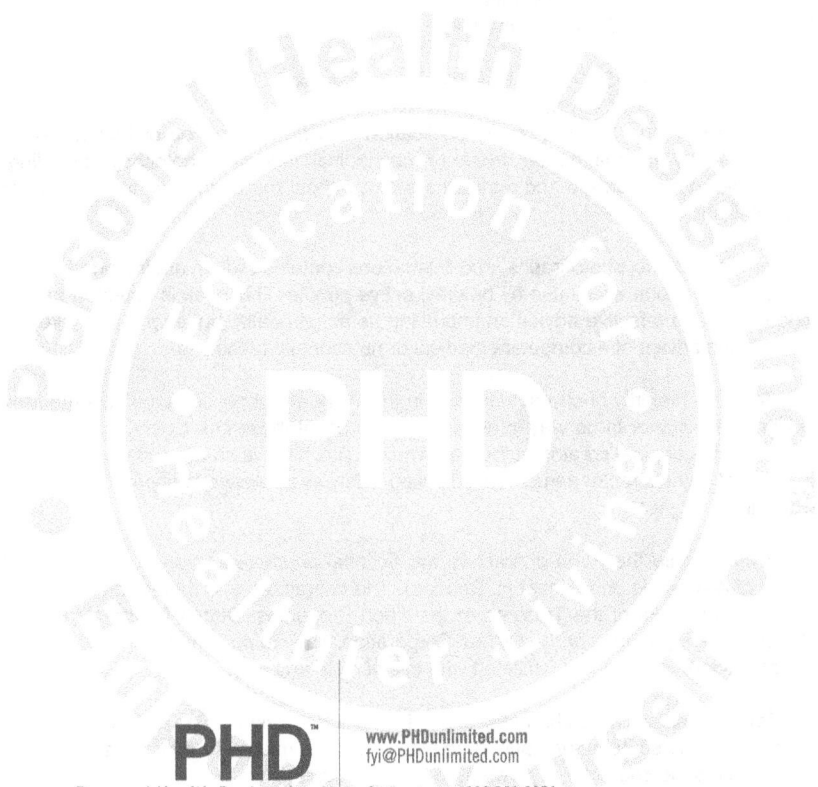

PHD™

Personal Health Design, Inc.

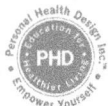

www.PHDunlimited.com
fyi@PHDunlimited.com

Corporate 602.321.8251
Fax 602.532.7505

FLORIDA	Boca Raton
	Hollywood
	Miami
CALIFORNIA	Santa Monica
	Beverly Hills
	San Diego
NEW YORK	Manhattan
	Brooklyn
ILLINOIS	Chicago
ARIZONA	Scottsdale

Health Designed with YOU in mind

A HEALTHIER EVER AFTER

CONTENTS

Foreword

"Did you remember to take your vitamins today?"

Most often, I guess that would be a parent speaking to their child, but not me, not lately. After being a teacher for about 35 years, it seems that the roles have been switched on me. I have become the student, at least when it comes to taking better care of myself.

When my son first told me he wanted to be a doctor, I was very proud. I envisioned him in his white coat and stethoscope, walking through hospital or running a big clinic. I knew he would be a good physician, helping people, always putting others first, supporting them and making them feel better. There were times when he was talking about health, so excited, it seemed he would never stop talking. Little did I know then that he would find his passion, teaching of all things, getting on a stage, or in front of a group of people in a small health food store, answering health questions and talking about healthier lifestyle choices.

I guess it wasn't a really big surprise when he told me he was planning on doing something a little different. First was the decision to go into an alternative medical program to study naturopathic medicine. He explained how he wanted to help educate people about healthier living before they were sick, demystifying how the body worked and how to maintain a healthy lifestyle. Although this approach was not as popular as it is today, his concept seemed rational.

After graduating, when I thought he was going to open an office, he told me he was going to culinary school and study healing with food. "Everybody eats", he said, "what you eat, when you eat, why you eat, etc. plays a major role in a person's health." Thinking about how much food impacts our lives each day, this idea made a lot of sense as well. I love my child and had no choice to support him.

"Did you know the root of the word doctor means to teach?" he asked me one day. He noticed that people wanted to know more, but health, and healthy living, is obviously a complex subject. He enjoyed making recommendations on how to live a little better, sharing tips to improve stress management and ways to make better nutrition choices. He was teaching, advising in a way that people of all ages could comprehend, and more important, apply the lesson to their personal lifestyle. Within my own family, including my husband and I, it has been great watching his younger brother, Kevin, learn how to make better choices for his health, while still maintaining his own identity and lifestyle.

In his lectures, my son, "Doc Rob", started using some stores from childhood, and characters from books I used to read to him at bedtime, in order to introduce some important health subjects to his audience. Perhaps a bit ironic, but once again, his story-telling approach, although maybe unconventional, seemed to work. I think he got that from his father.

Sure, the lessons or morals being introduced are a bit different from those fairy tales and children's stories, and he may mix in a movie reference from the '80s, but still, the message is definitely clear. Although I have learned a lot from him over the years, I found his book to be full or rational information, easily comprehensible, and delivered in a style that worked for me. I must admit, I may be a little bit biased. Of course, I suggest you read it and come to your own conclusion. Enjoy the book and live a healthier ever after.

- A loving mother, supporting parent, and last but not least, a proud fellow teacher

Acknowledgments

A friend once told me that in life you end up with two families; your "blood" family and your "life" family. The first family you are born with, connected from birth whether you like it or not. The latter, your life family, are those people who you share a connection with more by choice or circumstance. Of course both families are important, and can vary greatly in size. To make mention of every individual would take up way too many pages. I am very grateful for both, and would like to take this opportunity to acknowledge some individuals and/or groups who have supported me, specifically with regard to this book. This is not the end, rather just the beginning... I am thankful from the bottom of my heart.

My parents, Helen & Mark; my brother Kevin and my "other" brother, Marlon and his family; Grandparents: Sylvia (Bubby) & Irving (Zayde) Badner & Elaine & Stanley Streisfeld; uncles and aunts (Victor, Harvey, Frieda, Kathleen), cousins, and those special families who have taken me in, maybe gave me a bed, a ride, or shared a meal... treating me like a son. Michelle & David Cohen, all their dogs who have shown me unconditional love, and of course, my man Joe.

All my friends who have let me crash on their couch or in the guest room, maybe not knowing or understanding what I was doing, but believed in me nonetheless. Helping me earn the nickname the "Nomadic Naturopath", perhaps they just lent me their ear for a bit while I rambled my idealistic vision of a healthier ever after for all.

(In no particular order, and not meaning to leave anyone out) Scott S., Cara G., Bryan C., Chris C., Chris G., Josh K., Evan C., Nigel W., Cara B., Celina H., Mike H., Alex R., Amanda P., Lance H., Billy

O., Glen and Carrie G., Anna O., Lawrence C., Jessica E., Christie D., Jessica A., Nathan H., Becka K., Allison & Gary, Elena, Sasha, Inga, Lauren, Dory, Franceska & Ilonka, Dan T., Sabrina C., Robin A., Fernando V., Melissa K., Ulle L., Linda & Mike, Roman M., Jenn W., Eileen M., Richard P., Jeremy, Sonya F., Danielle K., Lindsey and the rest of the Wolf Pack, the Sarnoffs, the Wassermans, the Gordons, the Zalcburgs, the Kaufmans, the Shawns, and all those great reps in the Natural Products Industry (you know who you are).

There are many professors, colleagues, healers, teachers, co-workers, etc., who whether or not they knew it or might want to admit it, impacted my life to this point; acting as guides or mentors, helping to plant the seeds which helped me gain the understanding of healthier living, hopefully communicated in this book.

Professor Paul Naamon, Dr. James Sensenig, Donna Gates, Dr. Carlos Santo, Dr. Michael Reed, Dr. Decker Weiss, Jordan Rubin, Selina Delangre, Jill Turner, Jason Mitchell, Anne Marie Colbin (and the Natural Gourmet Crew), Sally Fallon, Ken Gootkind, Lynn Gordon, Maggie, Audra C., Dr. P Mittman, Joanna Hagen, Dr. Ginger Southall, Dr. Susan Hunt, Dr. Peter Wannigman, Dr. Jordan Steinberg, Dr. David Blyweiss, Dr. Alex Coracides, Dr. Jesse Haggard, The Paxsons, Frank Guzzo, Dr. Jon Crowfoot, Tom Bohager, Theo Quinto, Harmony and family, and Kerry Jacobson.

Special recognition for this book goes to:

Dr. Samantha Slotnick for creative, editorial, and emotional support,
Jason Love for humor advice and the "Snapshots",
Hilary Gerber for research support,
Nathalie Strassburg for layout, formatting, and design,
John Bindrum for the really great book cover, &
Stacey Weckstein for believing when others doubted, and for your constant love and support.

Finally, I feel it is important to acknowledge all of the people who support good causes and organizations, like Patch Adams' Gesundheit Hospital Project (www.patchadams.org), and all those who share in the vision, belief, and commitment of a healthier ever after for all.

THANK YOU!

All the best in health and happiness,

Doc

Rob

Introduction

Once upon a time, fairy tales and nursery rhymes painted vivid pictures of happily-ever-after, and the promise of a bright future. We were swept away, as children, by dreams of happily ever after, and enchanted by the magic of fairies and witches. But happily ever afters don't come from a fairy's magic wand—we have to make them ourselves. A magical life begins by taking personal responsibility for creating a healthy life, and making choices every day that lead us to feeling light and vibrant. *A Healthier Ever After* presents a path to a healthier, happier future.

Healthy living is a mindset. The choices we repeatedly make become our habits, and improving these habits takes a blend of motivation and education. *A Healthier Ever After* illustrates how each of us can create a mindset of health, learning new lessons from some old friends—a cast of characters borrowed from literary lore. Together, they demonstrate how our daily choices sculpt our health and the health of our families and our society. The time to set the right course is now—for yourself, for your loved ones, and for your children.

In this book, you will learn ways to achieve and maintain a healthy lifestyle from some favorite old characters. Hansel and Gretel will provide nutritional insights, and we will look to Peanuts' Pig Pen for a lesson on germs. We'll look at how Mother Goose's Peter Piper was building immune health with his peck of pickled peppers, and consider some children's nutritional issues by looking at Winnie the Pooh and friends. Humpty Dumpty's fall raises many questions, from why he fell in the first place to which side of the health industry wall (East or West) you might choose if you had a fall. Mary Poppins knew about natural medicines, and you'll learn what was in her bag of tricks. We also learn from cartoons, such as Wile E. Coyote and his Road Runner cravings.

We learn about enzymes from Goldilocks, who suffered carb crash in the bears' house, and join Little Miss Muffet for curds and whey. Jack Sprat who would eat no fat and his wife who'd eat no lean teach us about fats, good and bad, and balance. We'll go up the hill with Jack and Jill to see what's in that water, and who better to learn from about a sound night's sleep than the princess from The Princess and the Pea? The Old Woman Who Lived in a Shoe has a lot to say about overcrowding, as we branch out to look at the larger picture. Then we fly off into the future with The Jetsons. We end, of course, with Happily Ever After.

The moral of the story: Perfect health may be unattainable, but great health is achievable.

CHAPTER 1

~·//·~

Hansel & Gretel
Lost in the Woods

*"The difference between school and life? In school,
you're taught a lesson and then given a test. In life,
you're given a test that teaches you a lesson."*

- Tom Bodett

Hansel and Gretel, a brother and sister lost in the woods, stumble across a house made of gingerbread that is decorated with bright candy and gumdrops. Although they were nearly eaten by a witch, everything worked out in the end: "Then all anxiety was at an end, and they lived together in perfect happiness."

Sounds kind of sweet, doesn't it? They were the children of a poor woodcutter whose wife (the children's mother or stepmother, depending upon the edition) decided the best way to save some money was to "lose" the two children in the woods. In the end, she died of what seemed to be a severe case of evilness. Many critics believe the story was a commentary on the harsh cruelty of poverty in the Middle Ages and that it stemmed from actual instances of children being abandoned to fend for themselves. Are we, because of our own life circumstances, endangering our children when we leave them to fend for themselves in a fast food culture?

∾

THE AGE OF THE CONSCIOUS CONSUMER

Life is filled with challenges. Short of time, nutrition seems to be the first thing we sacrifice, for ourselves and for our children. Money is another factor that can easily guide a consumer's choice, and a fast food or canned meal is cheaper and easier than a fresh, organic meal.

3

Snapshots at jasonlove.com

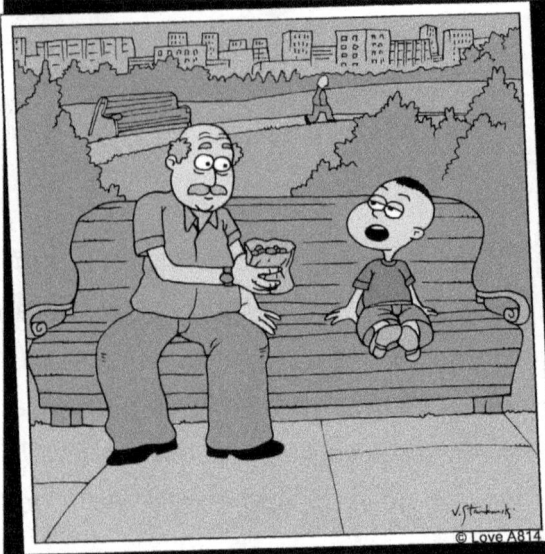

"I'm not allowed to take candy from strangers,
so, uh … tell me about yourself."

Packaged foods and quick fixes are easy when we're on the run and are easy to pack up for kids. But what are we sacrificing?

Sure, kids like colorful foods filled with sugar and additives, but we are the ones who choose what to buy. The more sugary snacks we give them, the more they crave sugar, and the more processed foods they eat, the less they appreciate the tastes of real, whole foods. An adult has, whether aware of it or not, a greater ability to make choices and to be more informed about food and health. Children trust in their parents to take care of them, to feed them properly, and to keep them healthy.

Like Hansel and Gretel, many children today are left "in the woods" to consume whatever is convenient or, even worse, what has been marketed to them through the media and commercials that sponsor their favorite cartoons. We can easily see why they would be so attracted to candy, fast food, soda, and other unhealthy "foods." Of

Conscious consumers make a difference and have affected the practices, labeling, and products offered by large corporations.

course they are drawn to the gingerbread house with gumdrops and candy canes when left on their own in the world of high-priced marketing campaigns.

Young children normally reject new foods the first time they try them. But most will accept a new food eventually and they should be offered the same food repeatedly with gentle encouragement.

In caring for our children, we need to educate them about how to make better choices when it comes to what they eat. No age is too young. Obesity, diabetes, and other health issues often begin in childhood. But the adult (or adults) in the household must first educate themselves about how to make healthy choices, so they can teach their children.

This level of personal responsibility in making choices is not only important for parents, but for everyone from the young to the "young at heart", and for those who want vibrant bodies and minds to keep pace! I am especially excited to share this information with young adults and teach them to make conscious, health affirming choices. After all, this is a generation poised to lead a movement of conscious consumerism by demanding fair and full labeling disclosure and letting those in the food and health industries know that consumers will ask questions and make informed choices.

Your body is creating itself every day, and the damaging effects of harmful foods can be cumulative. Making good dietary choices is an investment in a healthier ever after.

With all of the conflicting health information available and the number of illnesses and chronic problems linked to diet, conscious consumerism can make the difference between suffering chronic or recurrent health problems and living a rich, full, healthy life.

We have been living in The Chemical Age. In response, and for the sake of our health, this should become The Age of the Conscious Consumer.

> *Power is the faculty or capacity to act, the strength and potency to accomplish something. It is the vital energy to make choices and decisions. It also includes the capacity to overcome deeply embedded habits and to cultivate higher, more effective ones.*
>
> – Stephen R. Covey

THE ABUNDANCE CHALLENGE

For most of us, the challenge is not the lack of abundance, but overabundance. Before pesticides, diets were naturally rich with organic foods. Organic produce and products are more expensive, and pesticides allow farmers to grow more and sell for competitive prices, but we have to be careful about what we take into our bodies. A fast food hamburger may be less than a dollar, but what is the price to our bodies?

We have large supermarkets, grocery stores and restaurants with options and opportunities to eat pretty much whatever and whenever we want. We have to be conscious of and grateful for this modern privilege, but must also look back and hold onto what was good and nourishing to the body and soul. Our ancestors were most likely hunters and gatherers, early farmers, or fishermen who relied on nature in order to eat and to stay alive. People also had to depend more on family, neighbors, and community. Some would grow produce, others would raise cattle and supply dairy, and some others would make tools and equipment to be able to work the land better. Together, they turned the gifts of the land into hearty, life-sustaining meals. After the long, hard days of work, the family would sit down to eat, and be grateful for what they had, whether a lot or just a little.

Access to large quantities of cheap food makes it easy, but not advisable to choose quantity over quality. The truth is that when you choose quantity over quality, you're getting

> *Eating patterns in the toddler period set the framework for eating throughout childhood and later life.*

more food, but less nutrition. Choose quality for yourself and your family. It does take more time to prepare fresh foods, and they don't last as long as foods loaded with preservatives, but when you increase the quality in your nutrition, you will improve the quality of your life.

෬৯

SITTING DOWN TO EAT

Food is unifying. Everybody eats. Meals are a time to relax, whether alone or in the company of others. The sit-down meal has become all too rare with our fast-paced lives and the abundance of food we grab on the go. But arranging to share a meal may be the one point during the day that brings everyone in the family together. Laughing, sharing stories, taking time for ourselves and time with each other, these are all part of healthy living and the relationship with food and nourishment that we must not forget or neglect.

> Early on, children can regulate how much they eat, but not what they are offered.

But many of us don't take the time to sit down to eat, or even chew! Digestion will be better when you eat your meals sitting down, not while multi-tasking six other things. Chewing is important, too. Many people don't take the time to chew, which is actually the first part of the digestion process. Food is meant to begin breaking down in your mouth and is harder on the stomach if it doesn't, so give your stomach a break and chew!

෬৯

WHEN TO LET GO

As important as dietary concerns are and as much as you learn about being a conscious consumer, stressing out about eating perfectly can be counter productive to well being. Sometimes you really need to forget about calories, forget about whether its raw or organic, and just sit back with friends and/or family and enjoy the time together.

People often say to me, "I eat well six days of the week, and I have one cheat day where I pretty much eat whatever I want…all the bad stuff." I tell people they are harming themselves with this approach, and not because I think that doing this is bad for their health; but I would change the attitude and language they are using. I recommend restructuring the language and mindset to refer to this day as a treat day: a day to reward oneself for caring about health enough to make good, conscious choices the other six days of the week. Even if you don't choose the 6:1 ratio, it is important to keep a positive attitude and focus on all the good things you do for yourself. Maybe you don't go to the gym five days a week, but going three days is better than none. There have been times in my life where I felt I was "healthier," and periods where I wasn't making enough good choices. Health, like life, is always changing.

The more good choices you make as a conscious consumer, the more flexibility you have to indulge yourself on occasion. Health comes from not only your food choices, but your ability to enjoy life!

Your life is the sum result of all the choices you make, both consciously and unconsciously. If you can control the process of choosing, you can take control of all aspects of your life. You can find the freedom that comes from being in charge of yourself.
– Robert F. Bennett

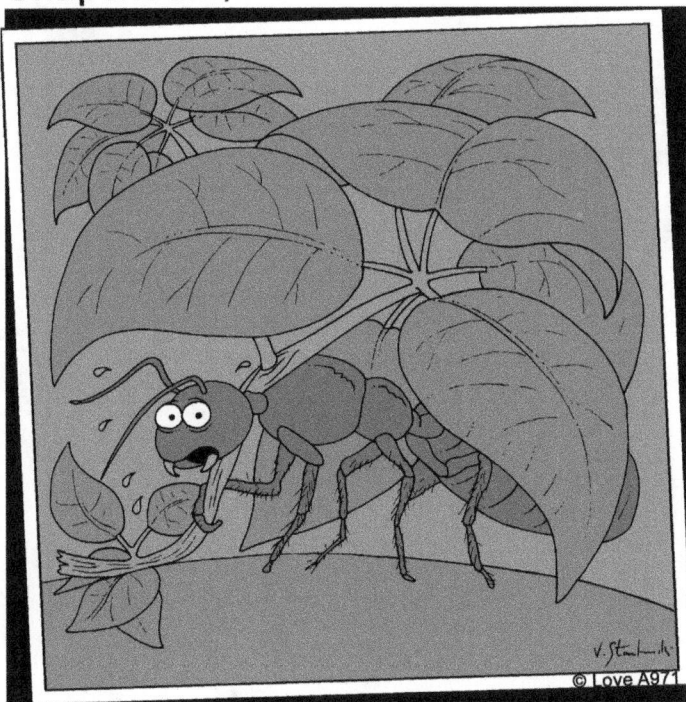

"High hopes nothin'. I've got kids to feed."

CHAPTER 2

※

Pig Pen
A Little Dirt Won't Hurt

"The supreme irony of life is that hardly anyone gets out of it alive." - Robert A. Heinlein

Remember Charlie Brown's friend, Pig Pen? He was always in the midst of a cloud of dust and dirt, and he seemed to take it all in stride. In fact, he referred to it proudly as "the dust of ancient civilizations," since he would go so long without washing it off. Even when he finally did, he was instantly dirty again. He was, as he admitted, a "dust magnet."

We are all, to a lesser degree of course, dust magnets. It is impossible to be completely clean of every last bit of microscopic dust or bacteria. You come in contact with billions of microorganisms every day. Just about every surface you touch, the air around you, your skin, your mouth, your digestive system, and even this book, are all covered in microscopic organisms. Microorganisms are, quite essentially, a fact of life.

~⌇9)

GET A LITTLE DIRTY

We don't have to go as far as Pig Pen, but a little dirt won't hurt. While hygiene is essential to good health, we have become too afraid of getting a little dirty. We use antibiotic hand sanitizers and sprays to wash away even the mere concept of a germ. As we take these measures and use these products as precautionary steps to protect health, we may instead experience the opposite effect. Constant use of antibacterial gels and cleansers actually weakens the body's immune system by not letting us get exposed. We also create super strains or mutant forms of bacteria, as they adapt to fight our ever-increasing strengths of anti-bacterial products and pharmaceuticals.

Children who grow up on farms have significantly fewer allergies and asthma than children growing up nearby but not exposed to the animals, bacteria and "dirt" on the farm.

Overuse of antimicrobials like triclosan (the active ingredient in antibacterial soaps) has been linked to resistant E. coli and salmonella bacteria; instead of protecting people from bad bugs, it made the bad bugs stronger!

At times, the sanitizer is more dangerous than a little dirt, containing chemicals, additives, and base ingredients that are more harmful than the dirt and microorganisms they were meant to fight. In one recent case, children were experiencing alcohol intoxication and liver damage from using alcohol-based hand sanitizers. When it is necessary to use sanitizing products, look for products with all natural ingredients.

೧෨

BAD BACTERIA

We actually have a micro-universe inside our digestive systems. There are a lot of friendly, good for you bacteria, but also some bad guys, parasites, yeast, fungi, etc. Often, when we are in a state of imbalance, the bad guys seem to survive and end up making matters worse. Even when you are exposed to certain not-so-friendly germs, your body's immune system is designed to jump to your aid and fight off the invader to protect you. Your immune system not only takes care of that microorganism, but also records the type of bacteria or virus it was into a database. That way, if you ever encounter the same critter again, your body is able to react even faster and fight more effectively. The body is pretty smart.

In our fear of all bacteria, we have created a state of attack on food before we consume it. We microwave, spray, and irradiate–yes, we actually douse food with radiation! We also kill the good bacteria in fighting bacterial infections when we take the antibiotics our doctors prescribe (and often over-prescribe). In doing these things, we harm ourselves and kill not only the bad bacteria, but also the good. We need

Cirradiated Food

Nearly all produce currently being imported to the US today is irradiated. In an effort to improve safety of imported food from unfriendly bacteria and organisms, we douse it with radiation, potentially harmful rays of energy. Irradiation affects the quality and safety of foods. A strong body of research shows that vitamins, nutrients, and essential fatty acids are destroyed during the process, while harmful free radicals and chemical by-products are produced. How can we avoid irradiated foods? The safest food is always fresh, local, and organic.

Source: http://www.citizen.org

to use healthier methods to fight bad bacteria, and we have to replace that good bacteria to maintain a healthy balance.

❧

"FRIENDLY" BACTERIA

Farmers used to reach down, pull a carrot or other vegetable from the ground, wipe it off and take a bite. There was actually good bacteria in the soil that the farmer consumed when eating the food. (Farming and agriculture have surely changed in recent times, and I do advise you clean your produce before consuming—especially if it is not organic—and avoid non-organic foods listed on page 17, in the "Dirty Dozen" box!) But we should remember that some bacteria are friendly to our bodies.

A healthy digestive system is maintained by beneficial bacteria. In fact, when dogs and cats get sick, they often go outside to eat some grass. Somehow, they "know" they need some good bacteria and to consume it from the soil. Animals often know instinctively what they need. Humans tend to be less "intelligent" in that way, so we gain our knowledge through research. We have discovered good bacteria called probiotics. (We're also not meant to eat dirt, so thankfully we can find our probiotic supplements in healthy foods and in products and supplements found at our local health food stores.)

Probiotics, which are gaining popularity in both supplement form (as

Not only does triclosan increase super bugs, but it also encourages widespread bacterial cross-resistance to certain antibiotics.

Excess "good hygiene" is linked to inflammatory bowel disease (IBD), and some scientists think that dogs and cats also get IBD when they are kept in unnaturally clean conditions.

capsules or powders) and in certain foods, such as yogurt, are essential for good digestive health and support a healthy immune system. In fact, even the name we give them shows their essential nature: "pro" means "for" and "biotics" means "life". Regardless of which product you choose, it is important to recognize the body's need for probiotics and to use them to restore and maintain health and balance. Probiotics are essential when regaining balance after taking antibiotics. They are also important for keeping that balance on a regular basis, as we are all compromised by stress and nutritional deficiencies.

∾

BEST DEFENSE

Pig Pen's Guide to Immunity

◇ Don't be afraid of good bacteria.

◇ Supplement your diet with probiotics (good bacteria) to maintain digestive health.

◇ Remember hygiene basics, but don't worry about a little dirt or be over-zealous about using antibacterial products.

◇ Have fun–even if it means getting a little dirty.

◇ They are also important for keeping that balance on a regular basis, as we are all compromised by stress and nutritional deficiencies. I recommend buying refrigerated probiotics that are shipped cold in glass bottles, use full-culture processing with "super strain" bacteria, and guarantee potency thru expiration date.

As always, the best defense is a strong immune system. It seems that we have become less confident in our immune system's ability to protect us from illness. The overuse of antibiotics, and the corresponding creation of powerful, mutant strains of bacteria haven't made health maintenance easy, but there are numerous ways to support our immune systems. Other ways include getting enough sleep, taking supplements, drinking enough clean water, and exercising regularly. These are all areas that are stressed throughout this book because so much of creating a "healthier ever after" depends on having a strong, healthy immune system.

The bacterial balance is important and Probiotics are essential for regaining that balance when lost. Another natural product that helps in regaining and maintaining balance is Silver Hydrosol, a natural germ-fighting liquid available in nearly all health food stores. Silver has long been known as a germ fighter. Our ancestors used bowls made from silver to keep food safe from bacteria. (More on Silver Hydrosol in Chapter 11, Jack and Jill.)

Keep your food and home as natural as possible. Even certain natural cleaning products now include probiotics in their formulas. These products are formulated not only to kill germs and bad bacteria, but to also leave good bacteria behind. I do not suggest you roll your baby around in a pile of dirt to be more like Pig Pen and certainly don't advocate eating dirt! However, it is important to consider that some exposure to nature's elements helps develop a stronger constitution. Relax just a little. Don't you remember the five-second rule?

Fermented foods also promote good bacteria and fight the bad. Read more about fermented foods in the next chapter, Peter Piper.

The Dirty Dozen   When to go organic!

Commonly known as the "dirty dozen," the following are the foods that contain the most chemicals. This list was compiled using FDA and the USDA tests from 100,000 samples of food. The pesticides found in these studies cause cancer, birth defects, nervous system and brain damage, and development problems in children.

1. Meat (beef, pork, poultry)
2. Dairy (milk, cheese, butter)
3. Strawberries
4. Apples
5. Tomatoes
6. Potatoes
7. Spinach (and other greens, including lettuce)
8. Coffee
9. Peaches and Nectarines
10. Grapes (especially imported)
11. Celery
12. Bell Peppers (Red & Green)

Source: http://www.reneeloux.com/go_organic/dirty_dozen.html

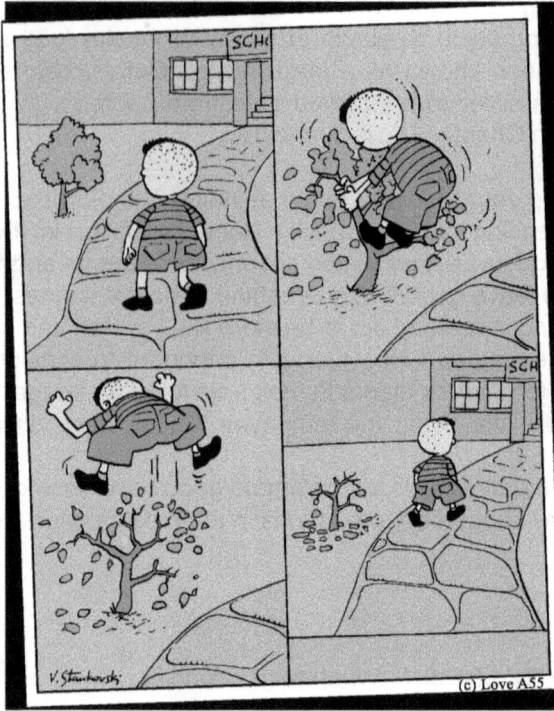

Every generation, our kinship with
nature slips a little further.

Notes

CHAPTER 3

Peter Piper
And the Virtues of Pickled Peppers

"Peter Piper picked a peck of pickled peppers. A peck of picked peppers Peter Piper picked. If Peter Piper picked a peck of pickled peppers, how many pickled peppers did Peter Piper pick?"

Of course, how can we have a book featuring children's tales without quoting the great Mother Goose? How many pecks of pickled peppers Peter Piper picked in this famous nursery rhyme is not as important as why he loved them so much. Pickling vegetables, a process also known as fermentation, has been part of food preparation for thousands of years. Remember, refrigerators are a relatively recent invention.

⌒♈

FERMENTATION

Fermentation refers to the growth of beneficial microorganisms, more widely known as probiotics, on common foods. Fermentation gradually changes the characteristics of the food through the action of enzymes, produced by the probiotic bacteria, molds and yeasts. Fermentation is also now being used in supplements to naturally prolong shelf stability and increase nutritional value and absorption. Fermentation is even gaining popularity in green health drinks. Even though we have probiotic supplements, and more and more products formulated to keep good levels of beneficial bacteria in the body, certain

Peter Piper's Guide to Preserving Your Health

✧ Incorporate some healthy fermented foods into your diet.

✧ Beware of high-sugar fermented foods.

✧ Experiment with some new, exotic fermented foods to keep things interesting and fun.

✧ Realize that pasteurization is a process that uses high heat to destroy bacteria, both good and bad.

fermented foods should also be incorporated into the diet. In many types of foods, especially soy, this enzymatic processing enhances the nutritional value, improves digestion, and promotes a healthy inner ecosystem.

You may have heard of functional foods. These are foods that have known health benefits and reduce the risk of disease. One important group of functional foods consists of those that are fermented. I call these FFFs: functional fermented foods. FFFs are an important part of a healthy diet.

FFFs have a long, healthy history of success. The explorers, who sailed uncharted seas in search of new lands full of treasure, would lose nearly all of their men from illness or malnutrition. Upon incorporating fermented foods in their diets, a kind of sauerkraut some say, the health of the sailors improved dramatically, and fewer died from malnourishment.

Fermented foods can be found in nearly every culture and civilization. Examples include kimchee, a form of fermented cabbage from Korea, that is a daily staple in nearly all Korean households. Kimchee production can be traced back nearly 3,000 years. Kefir, a fermented dairy product gaining recent popularity, originally comes from Turkey. The word actually means, "to feel good."

Many modern condiments, including ketchup and mustard, were originally fermented foods. Nowadays, however, they've been neutered to become strictly flavor enhancers. Miso, tempeh, and natto are all fermented soy foods, which have been staples in Japanese diets for centuries.

Sauerkraut, kombucha, pickles, vinegar, sourdough bread, and yogurt are all examples of fermented foods that can benefit

Natural vs. Unnatural Soy Products

Traditionally prepared soy sauce is made from soybeans that are mixed with roasted grain (usually wheat, rice, or barley) and fermented for several months. Once the aging process is complete, the mixture is strained and bottled. Synthetically manufactured soys are produced in a matter of days through a hydrolytic reaction and seasoned with corn syrup, caramel coloring, salt and water. These unnatural products lack not only the health benefits of traditional, naturally produced soy products, but the flavor, too. Sometimes, a slightly metallic taste can also be detected. Look for traditionally prepared varieties, preferably organic.

health and improve digestive health.

Vinegars can be a bit confusing as the choices are extensive and, while flavor may dictate choice, the quality and benefits of all vinegars are not equal. Some are filtered or processed. Others, such as balsamic, incorporate adding sugar into the fermentation process. These may taste sweet, but are not as healthy as, for instance, raw, unfiltered, unsweetened apple cider vinegar. Apple cider vinegar has been shown to help control yeast/Candida in the body and restore balance. (It's also great in salad dressings and other recipes!) A proper PH (balance of acid-alkaline) is important, especially if you are suffering from achy joints and muscles, recurrent yeast infections, poor digestion, and a number of other symptoms, which may or may not seem related. Apple cider vinegar may help...plus, it's safe and relatively inexpensive.

One of the foremost experts in fermented foods and nutrition is Donna Gates, author of *The Body Ecology Diet*. For over 20 years, Donna has been helping people all over the world regain their health. In the last five years she has been focusing in on the essential balance of bacteria found in the digestive system and has even used her knowledge of beneficial micro-flora to help prevent and reverse autism. Donna writes:

"To prevent autism and other childhood disorders I feel it is important to teach young mothers-to-be to eat plenty of fermented foods before and during their pregnancy, to build a strong immune system in their own body and in their baby's. Fermented foods are vital for very efficient digestion, which helps provide availability of nutrients that the mother-to-be and her baby need during the pregnancy. When the mother eats fermented foods, her birth canal becomes populated with beneficial micro-flora, the baby passes thru the birth canal, picks up the healthy micro-flora, and receives many benefits. Some of those benefits are:

• They always digest their food better which provides superior nutrition, especially in the early days as the brain and bones are developing. The micro-flora inside of us are highly intelligent beings and know what we need. They manufacture B Vitamins and Vitamin K right down inside of us so they can be quickly assimilated, passing quickly thru the gut wall. This is much more effective than taking a B Vitamin supplement because the micro-flora always know what B Vitamin to make and what we are lacking.

• Many babies today have trouble digesting their own mother's milk or formulas. When they have plenty of healthy micro-flora living inside the intestines, this won't be a problem.

• Micro-flora help the baby have a healthy immune system and the child is less likely to have problems like ear infections or have the need for antibiotics.

While 1 in 94 boys are now autistic, this epidemic is just one of many affecting our children today. Childhood obesity, diabetes, ADHD, and even cancer are serious concerns.

Beneficial micro-flora, however, found in a "probiotic diet" like Body Ecology's, and discussed here in this book, is really for people of all ages – from the prenatal years until we draw our last breath."

Apple Cider Vinegar

When the body is too acidic, try taking a small shot of apple cider vinegar (between a teaspoon and tablespoon) in an 8 oz glass of water. Take it before bed and/or first thing in the morning. Warm or room temperature is best. Squeezing fresh lemon and adding some mineral-rich sea salt (to taste) to a glass of water is also a good option. Also, try these other ways to increase the body's alkaline level:

◈ Have a cup of miso soup (a functional fermented food)
◈ Increase your mineral intake.
◈ Increase green foods in your diet.
◈ Decrease animal proteins in your diet.
◈ Increase fruit and vegetable consumption.

Apple Cider Vinegar Dressing

Mix 1 cup of raw, unfiltered, apple cider vinegar with 1/4 cup of raw honey, 1.5 cups of extra virgin olive oil, and a dash of sea salt. Shake well before each use! Feel free to experiment with your favorite spices. For extra flavor and health, add a dash of cayenne pepper.

To learn more:

"The Body Ecology Diet, 10th Ed.", Donna Gates, BED Publications, 2007 www.bodyecology.com

"Truly Cultured": Rejuvenating Taste, Health and Community with Naturally Fermented Foods, Nancy Lee Bentley, Two Pie Radians Foundation, 2008 www.trulycultured.com

"Wild Fermentation": The Flavor, Nutrition, and Craft of Live-Culture Foods, Sandor Ellix Katz, Chelsea Green Publishing, Co, 2003 www.wildfermentation.com

Snapshots at jasonlove.com

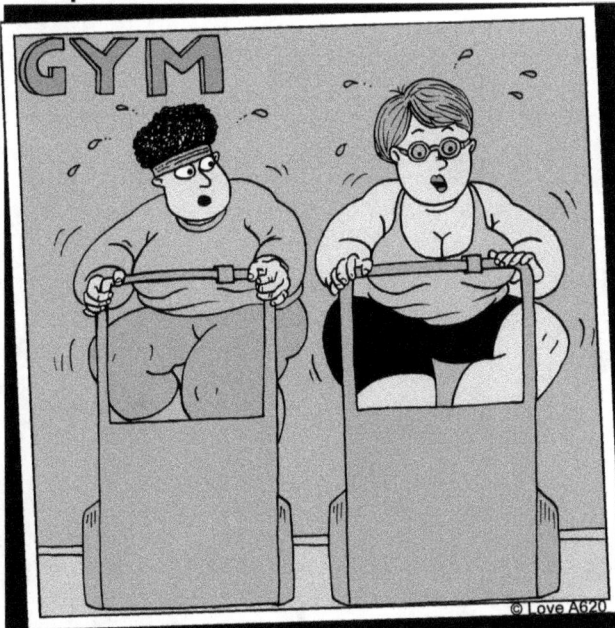

"If you had a tapeworm, would you keep it?"

CHAPTER 4

❧

Winnie The Pooh
Stuck on Sugar

I*f you live to be 100, I hope I live to be 100 minus one day so I never have to live without you."—Winnie the Pooh*

As we get older and our jobs and responsibilities overtake our days, playtime with childhood friends seems so long ago. Whether it was little league, hide and go seek, or maybe sharing snacks after school, your experiences with friends were foundational to the lessons you learned and probably influenced the type of person you are today. Winnie the Pooh and friends are a diverse little bunch who are there for each other, though each one has a shortcoming or two (as we all do). But looking at them from a nutritional perspective, I have some suspicions about their diets (beyond, of course, Winnie's obvious attachment to honey).

❧

CHILDREN'S HEALTH ISSUES

So many children's health issues come from the foods they eat. Looking at Pooh, Tigger and Eeyore, we can see a few common issues and how they affect the personalities and outlooks of these characters… and our children.

Winnie the Pooh

First let's look at our friend, Pooh, whose belly sticks out of his little red shirt. Pooh is the sugar loving candy craving kid who doesn't know when to stop, even when he gets his rear stuck in a tree while going after some honey. Was it his high-sugar diet, lack of exercise, and larger-than-average

> **A**fter the age of three, overweight children are eight times as likely to become overweight adults.

portion size? Each factor plays a role in obesity and health issues.

We have, in this country, an epidemic of obese children. Obesity numbers in children in the US, and around most of the world are growing at a fast rate. Results of high-sugar low-nutrient diets are obesity, diabetes, autoimmune disorders, and frequent, severe colds.

Tigger

Then of course there's Tigger. Bouncing all around, unable to sit still. He's too young to be cranked up on Starbucks, but something has the fun-loving friend of Pooh hyperactive and out of control. Tigger would likely be one of the growing number of our children being diagnosed with ADD (Attention Deficit Disorder) and ADHD (Attention Deficit Hyperactivity Disorder), or some other "disease" state.

Current medical treatments lean heavily on pharmacology, which requires naming and treating "diseases" based on behaviors and attention problems, which may result from simple food allergies or bad nutritional choices. In fact, when a child is diagnosed with a hyperactive disorder, some schools are mandating that drugs be administered to the students, or the school may choose to not allow the student into class. Chemical sweeteners and additives in common foods and beverages and exposure to a toxic environment are often at the root of attention problems. If they are not the cause, they are often contributing factors, which should be eliminated or reduced. Equally detrimental is allowing kids to live in front of the TV or play video games for far too many hours each day. Some games are fine, even educational, and there is nothing wrong with having some fun— but balance, time outdoors, and time interacting socially with friends and family are all important considerations for raising healthy, happy, well-balanced kids.

The guidelines for diagnosing ADD and ADHD are based on symptoms, but give little attention to the individual and his or her environment and diet. Again, this is not to say that drugs are all bad, but there has to be a reason why so many children are hyperactive, unable to concentrate, or expressing behavioral problems. Food is meant to nourish us. However, it is often overlooked in favor of pharmaceuticals. There is more money to be made in selling drugs than in selling good, organic food–and pharma companies know that starting young builds an enormous customer base!

Some literature suggests that the average American senior (65 and over) takes over 30 different prescriptions. The average number of prescriptions per senior rose from 19.6 in 1992 to 28.5 in 2000 (a 45% increase) and is projected to continue rising to 38.5 in 2010. That will be an increase of 96% from 1992!

Number of Prescriptions for Seniors 1992-2005 & Projected for 2010

Year	Number of Prescriptions per Senior
1992	19.6
1994	20.7
1996	22.6
1998	26.5
2000	28.5
2005	34.4
2010	38.5

Source: Data compiled by PRIME Institute for Families USA

Never too young to start?

Even in Elementary school, Big Pharma is gaining a larger and larger customer base. Perhaps if children take fewer drugs, they will need fewer when they get older. Novel thought, I know.

It has become easier to label a bunch of symptoms, (or in this case, personality/behavioral issues) as "diseases," rather than encourage and educate patients to restore balance through nutrition.

Once children take medications, several new problems arise. First, it is very difficult to get them off the drugs; second, they have to deal with new secondary problems from side effects; and third (but of no less importance), the label of having that "disease" or condition sticks with them. What if a history of ADD in school affects admission decisions for college or in the work place? Maybe beginning with healthy, conscious choices such as more fruits and vegetables, whole food supplements, fewer processed foods, higher quality food ingredients, exercise, and other nourishing lifestyle choices are worth the effort in the long run.

> Children with gastrointestinal problems are at risk for further deficiencies due to malabsorption.

Eeyore

And then there is Eeyore. I can almost hear you thinking, "No, don't pick on poor Eeyore." Well, I am not picking on the poor guy, but something has him pretty down. He is clearly depressed, maybe suffering from food reactions or allergies.

Depression is becoming more and more of a problem for both children and adults. Again the use of drugs and pharmacology seem to be the first line of treatment, but a change in diet and some conscious choices might make all the difference.

Depression affects about 12.2 million women (1 in 5) and over 6 million men (1 in 10) each year in the United States. [1] Even those who don't suffer from chronic depression could use a little mood elevation now and then.

Quick Tips for Mood Elevation

1.   Consume food that nourishes the brain. Brain food includes organic free-range eggs and fresh, wild caught fish. High-quality fats contain mood-elevating benefits. These can also be found in supplements such as flax seed oil, fish oil, and cod liver oil. Research shows that people who take cod liver oil every day have significantly less depression than those who don't.

---

[1] Source: http://www.stress.org

2.   Exercise regularly, practice deep breathing, and try to meditate often. Endorphins (good neuro chemicals) are released when you exercise, elevating your mood and helping you feel well.

3.   Replace table salt with Celtic Brand® Sea Salt, which is not only a natural, healthy source of lithium (used to treat depression) but a great source of numerous minerals that help keep the body balanced.

4.   Make sure to socialize. Get out of the house or have a dinner party. Remember to CELEBRATE LIFE!!

‹∾⌯)

GUT REACTIONS

Why are obesity, attention deficit disorders, and depression so common in children? What is the common thread? Modern science loves to classify new diseases and conditions based on grouping symptoms. What if nearly all dis-ease in the body begins with what we consume and how our bodies react to it? Identifying the underlying cause and understanding the role and status of both internal and external environments is the beginning of a thorough, holistic approach to healing. Treatments that are aimed only toward easing or treating the symptoms don't address the underlying causes.

When our children get sick, sometimes chronically, we need to remember that many illnesses start right in their little (or like in Pooh's case, not so little) bellies. Again, the imbalance of the delicate environment in the digestive system is most often the beginning of dis-ease in the body. For instance, neurotransmitters–the little chemical messengers that send signals to the

> **E**ven in adolescence, what the mother eats, how often food is prepared at home, and what kinds of foods are available at home strongly influence what young people eat.

brain for depression, anxiety, and help regulate sleep patterns–are produced in the body's digestive system with the help of those good bacteria. Think of dominos. That small symptom, an earache or bellyache, is the first domino. Treating the symptom without finding out the cause will result in a cascade of other problems in the body if the root cause is not found and addressed.

Constant earaches, little skin rashes, recurrent stomachaches, etc., may seem like minor irritations, but what if they soon developed into Type 2 diabetes, ADHD, autism, or depression? A "sudden" illness may not be as sudden as we think. Often, little symptoms are signs of larger issues developing. Simply treating recurrent problems with creams and medicines without considering the cause may allow a small problem to develop into something more serious over time. In the next chapter, Humpty Dumpty, we'll take a closer look into the importance of prevention. It's important to determine the underlying cause of disease in the body, especially when many of these conditions can be traced back to the health of the digestive tract.

Illnesses are different for everyone, and causes can include diet, emotional health, family/home environment, and overly prescribed pharmaceuticals, to name a few. It would be foolish to assume that the answers to everyone's illnesses are exactly the same—but many issues do begin with a problem in the gut. This adds new meaning to the saying: *Never underestimate a gut reaction!*

> Good bacteria are the basis for a useful and safe treatment for diarrhea in children, which can be dangerous, even deadly. (Zinc supplementation can also treat and prevent diarrhea in children.)

Snapshots at jasonlove.com

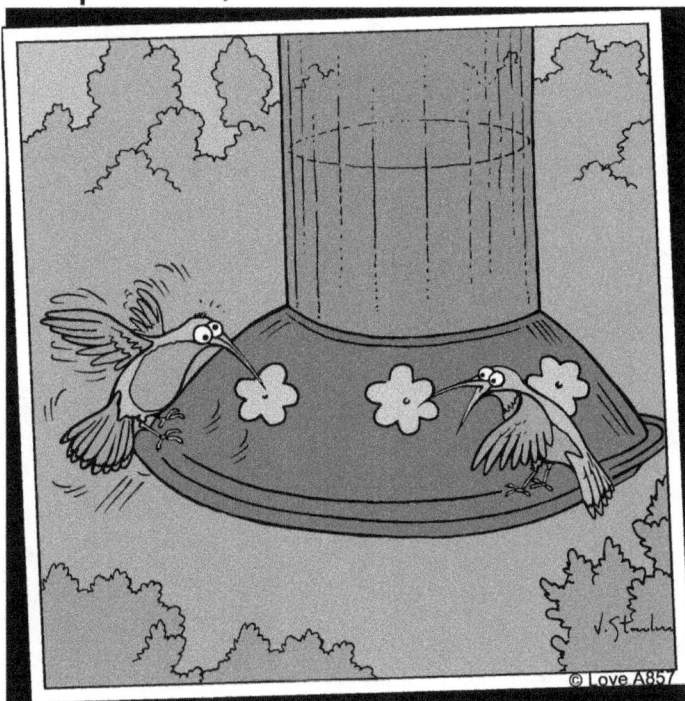

"Hey, uh, maybe you oughta take
a break from the sugar water."

CHAPTER 5

Humpty Dumpty
On the East / West Divide

"The best years of your life are the ones in which you decide your problems are your own. You do not blame them on your mother, the ecology, or the president. You realize that you control your own destiny." - Albert Ellis

*P*oor Humpty Dumpty, sitting around on a wall and down he falls. All the king's men (and–umm–their horses) couldn't put the poor guy back together again.

Our modern-day Humpty might be sitting on a couch or in an office chair, snacking on fast food and guzzling soda, coffee, or energy drinks just to make it through the day. When he falls down, all the top specialists still can't always put him back together again.

Modern technology and enhanced emergency procedures have made amazing leaps in the ability to save lives, and might have been able to save Mr. Dumpty. Today this field of medicine is more accurately referred to as "traumatic care" or "heroic medicine." But what about before we get to the point of needing "heroic medicine"? Who is your doctor or other healthcare provider? This person's philosophy affects your healthcare treatment, so understanding this will help you choose the right person for you and know when and where to get a second opinion.

⊙

MEDICAL CHOICES

If you're sitting up on the wall like Humpty and you need a doctor, which side of the wall will you choose—west or east?

West

Allopathic medicine (our traditional US healthcare system), also known as Western medicine, focuses on surgery and pharmacology in an effort to "fix" individuals and their symptoms. Traditionally, allopathic medicine treats symptoms. If you have a rash, you need a cream. If you have gas, you need a pill. The concern with over medicating (or medicating instead of making dietary or lifestyle changes) is that the problem doesn't go away. It is only suppressed, or masked. And now you're giving your body more chemicals to deal with, and you may have side effects on top of your original problems.

Frequent use of antibiotics, pharmaceuticals, excessive alcohol, and high-sugar diets stress the body and weaken the overall health of the digestive lining, wiping out the important bacteria that produce enzymes and help break down food. (See "Drug Warnings" later in this chapter for more details on the trouble with over-prescribing antibiotics.)

> **80%** of the developing world uses traditional herbal medicine as their primary method of healing.

East

Complementary and alternative medicine offer options that are alternatives to our traditional allopathic system. Many of the disciplines within the alternative health care field are referred to as "Eastern" medicine, because many of their philosophical roots can be traced back to ancient cultures, mainly Asian and Indian systems of healing, which are thousands of years old. On this side of the wall is a more holistic, natural approach to healing. "Alternative" medicine is concerned not only with healing, but with preventative care and strengthening the immune system. It is called "holistic" because it takes into account the "whole person." If you have a skin rash, for example, instead of giving you ointment for your skin (or in addition), a holistic practitioner will look at what you are putting into or in contact with your body to cause that reaction.

Naturopathic medicine, for instance, looks to treat the whole person naturally. The emphasis is not just on the symptoms, but also on using an integrative approach to finding the underlying cause of dis-ease. Many practitioners work with patients who also see Western, or allopathic, medical doctors, and might refer patients for tests to help identify a trouble spot or an acute condition.

Choice and Integration

Is one type of medicine good and the other bad? Although some professionals from both sides may feel that way, more and more consumers, as well as many health providers, actually want to integrate the two. Many traditional hospitals are integrating certain alternative practitioners into their treatment programs. In the best of both worlds, we identify the best healing methods, products, treatments and therapies from both sides of the wall. I call this "modern health."

༄♪

PREVENTION

---

*T*rials, temptations, and disappointments—all these help instead of hinder, if one uses them rightly. They not only test the fiber of a character, but strengthen it...Every trial endured and weathered in the right spirit makes a soul nobler and stronger than it was before.
- James Buckham

Imagine throwing a big rock into a quiet pond. Long after the rock is deep under the surface, the ripples are still spreading throughout the body of water. The ripples go out from the center and hit the shores in different locations. It's easy to sit on the shore and see the water come in, but we need to find the place where the ripples began. When discussing something like throwing rocks in a pond, where the ripples originate does not seem too important. But what if they become waves, eroding the shore on which your house is built, putting your home in jeopardy. You'd want to stop those ripples at the source if you could!

Now imagine that the waves hitting the shore represent symptoms of illness or imbalance in your body. A skin rash, a headache, chronic fatigue, graying hair, heartburn, or any other common or not-so-common symptom might seem like ripples, as small as those of a rock thrown into a pond. You may not consider them a big deal, and yes, it's easy to take a pill or apply a cream to address the immediate symptom, but it is also important to research and understand the underlying cause of the problem. Ignoring the symptoms may lead to something much more serious. Find the cause before your house begins to crumble into the sea.

A practitioner interested in preventative medicine might ask Mr. Dumpty what he was doing on the wall in the first place. What was he eating, doing, or experiencing that made him out of balance? A conscious consumer makes nutritional and lifestyle choices that are preventative of illness or harm–from exercise, to diet, to stress reduction. A good health care practitioner can help you with this and guide you in the right direction. Alternative therapies are, by nature, focused on prevention. However, many allopathic practitioners now focus on prevention, as well. And we all know that good exercise, diet, and lifestyle choices are important for staying healthy.

Exercise

Even if doctors can put Humpty back on the wall again, how long will he be okay if he just sits around on that wall all day? He needs to get "off the bench" and start playing the game. It is important to incorporate more exercise into your lifestyle, and make it something you enjoy doing. If running on a treadmill makes you miserable, then try swimming, playing tennis, or finding a basketball game in your neighborhood. If you can't find one, get some friends together and make it a regular thing. Some people love running, and others like lifting weights. Maybe you would enjoy dance classes. Obviously, factors like where you live, your schedule, your age and current health play a role in the types of exercise you choose.

Regular, light exercise, such as walking, can help maintain good health.

One form of exercise to consider, if you haven't already, is yoga. People of all ages have been grabbing their mats and heading off to the nearest yoga studio. Of course you can practice yoga in the quiet of your own home, but regardless of location, the benefits of yoga are apparent, and can be found on the following page.

SNAPSHOTS at jasonlove.com

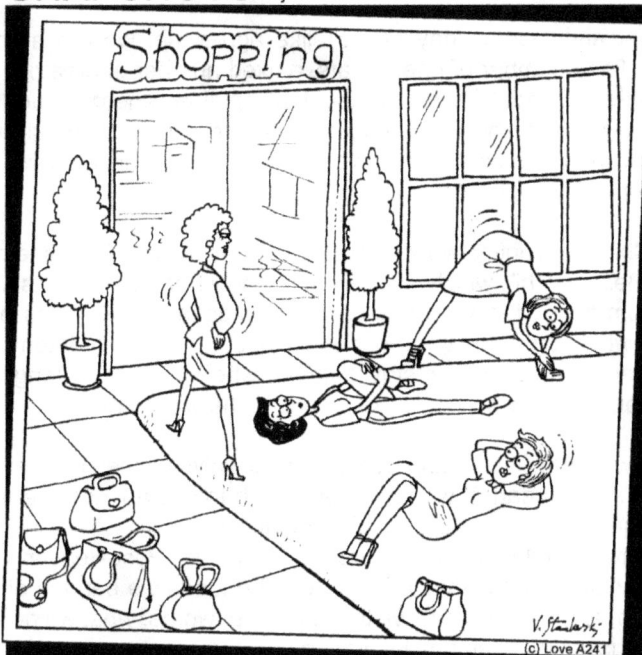

Serious shoppers stretch before taking on the mall.

Weight training offers many styles and techniques, just as yoga comes in many forms. One approach that I find interesting is called "functional fitness." Good for people of all ages, functional fitness utilizes stretch bands, medicine balls, and machines, focusing on movements which are in line with daily activities.

Two individuals in the fitness field who have impressed me with their philosophies and solid approaches to exercise are John Davies, founder and creator of Renegade Training (http://www. renegadetraining.com), and Juan Carlos ("JC") Santana, Director and CEO of the Institute of Human Performance (http://www.ihpfit.com). Both have elevated the art of exercise and fitness training.

Benefits of Yoga

The best time to plant a seed and grow a tree was twenty years ago; the second best time is now. - Ancient Chinese Proverb

Ancient and modern day sages alike agree that we are all born with a finite number of heart beats, a fixed number of breaths, and a relatively predetermined amount of spiritual energy. Such life force as termed 'chi', or 'prana', is considered by traditional healing arts the very essence of who we are, that which animates us, and without which we cease to exist.

The Chinese identify two sources of this vital energy. One is termed "Pre-Heaven Chi", which is received not only from our parents' DNA but from the collective message of up to seven generations past. Many would term this to be our constitution, that which determines whether we get sick or stay healthy, whether we live long and prosper, or wither and fade like leaves in the wintertime.

While we have little control over how well we've chosen our parents (no less our lineage), we have very much to say about the energy we acquire (or waste) as a result of our lifestyle habits. The ancients would refer to this second source of vitality as "Post-Heaven Chi", or the vital substance we extract from the foods we eat, the air we breathe, and the thoughts we think. In other words, what we do with the cards we've been dealt is very much in our own hands.

We in the western world view exercise in a manner reminiscent of how we live our lives as a society. That is, the harder we work, the more sweat we produce, the more grueling our efforts, the greater the reward. But is the "no pain, no gain" mantra truly within our best interest to continue to pursue? Is it possible that we are much more than the sum of our cardiac output, our flexibility, our bench press poundage, or our waist-to-hip ratio?

Yoga is by nature a restorative activity. Sanskrit for "union", the focus of yoga practice is to unite us with something greater than ourselves, be it God, spirit, or infinite consciousness. In fact, eight limbs of yoga actually exist and only one of those limbs involves the physical practice we've come to know as yoga. The remaining seven limbs focus on concepts such as "right living", "right mindfulness", and "purification", as steps toward greater connection with our higher self.

When we are engaged in the physical 'asana', or postural practice of yoga, our movements are intimately linked with our breath. The concept of 'pranayama', or breath control, is the very crux of what separates yoga from other forms of activity. In most any physical action, be it a planned workout or a simple walk up several flights of stairs, our breathing is re-active. That is to say, the harder we work, the faster and deeper we breathe. In true yoga practice, the opposite effect is sought. In short, we never move faster or work harder than our breath can sustain us, else we risk moving out of connection with our focus and practice. Are we limiting ourselves you might ask? Shouldn't we be working harder in pursuit of an ever more fit heart, tighter thighs, and slimmer waistline?

To maintain congruence between breath and movement means to be in integrity with our practice, a process that asks us to be fully present while engaged on our yoga mat. The rhythm of transition from posture to posture is fueled by steep and steady breathing, while every system of the body is called into action in a manner that replenishes, rather than depletes, our energy. We understand that we are tapped in to a universal energy much greater than ourselves, where our vitality reflects a state of optimal wellness on all levels - mind, body, and spirit.

The ancient practice of yoga is truly the perfect tool to address many of the challenges we face in our disease-based health care system. From its ability to lower blood pressure, reduce anxiety, shave body fat, to the benefits it offers to the health of our bones, joints, and muscles as well, yoga is a practice that should be in everyone's virtual medicine cabinet.

Dr. Carlos Santo is a licensed naturopathic physician and acupuncturist practicing in Scottsdale, Arizona. In addition to working with Personal Health Design and Doc Rob, he writes regular pieces for a web-based life coaching program called Tools to Life, is a certified yoga instructor, and teaches at the prestigious At One Yoga studio of Scottsdale.

SYNDROME X

Syndrome X is also known as metabolic syndrome. Sounds serious, right? Well, it must be! This "disease" is common in adults, but is now popping up in teens and children. The truth is, the term is used to describe a multitude of imbalances: blood sugar imbalances, Type 2 diabetes, achy joints, arthritis and inflammation, poor digestion, obesity, high cholesterol, low energy, gallstones, high blood pressure, infertility, hair loss, etc. Any of these sound familiar? There are so many different symptoms and signs of imbalance that the medical system has a hard time putting a label on it. They don't know which pill to prescribe first because they aren't sure where to start putting out the fires. Many now recommend diet and lifestyle changes. Doesn't it make more sense to make those changes before getting labeled?

Diet

Remember when you were able to eat just about anything—without it affecting your stomach? Like many, I had an iron stomach when I was younger. But somewhere along the line, the ability to digest became compromised and some things just didn't "agree" with us. This might change because of an overuse of antibiotics or years of processed foods, filled with preservatives, chemicals, high sugar, bad oils—all "nuked" to perfection in the microwave. The number of allergies suffered by infants, children, and adults is steadily rising. Lack of energy, chronic fatigue, even loss of libido could all be related, stemming from borderline malnourishment. Or maybe it was the fact that our lives had simply become more stressful and our bodies are struggling to handle it all. Maybe it's the quality of the foods and the environment. Diet is the focal point of *A Healthier Ever After* because a balanced, healthy diet is essential for preventing disease and maintaining overall health.

Lifestyle

We all have different lifestyles; we express ourselves in many ways—from hairstyles to clothes to the foods we eat. Many of us have dietary needs, restrictions, and preferences that become part of our identities. Your co-workers might not recognize you in the afternoon without your latte or candy bar. Maybe you're a "veggie" or a "health

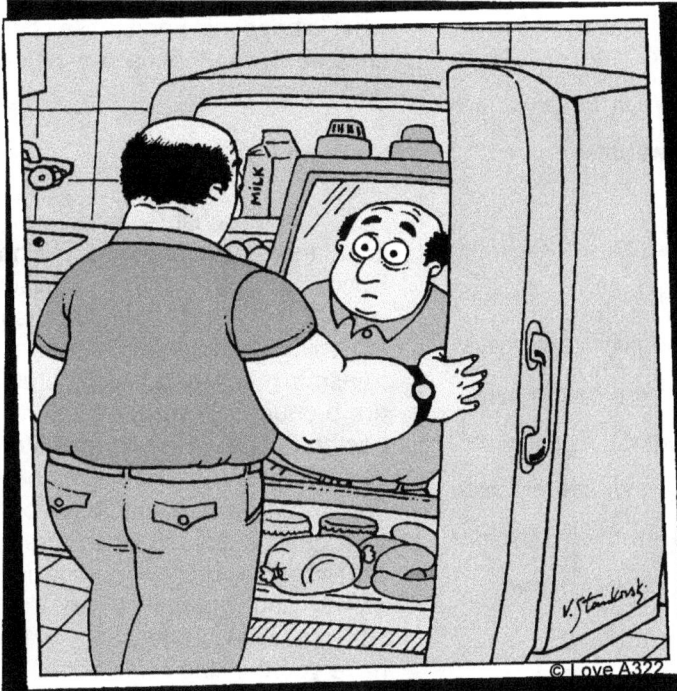

Bob devises the ultimate weight-loss system.

nut" or a "fast food junkie." Making even relatively small changes in how you approach each day will alter not only your personal style (maybe even earn you a new nick name), but also your life style. How often do we stop to realize we have fallen out of balance? Even when we do, and want to change our ways, it is typical to feel overwhelmed or helpless to actually do anything about it.

Are we just lazy? Perhaps, but if apathy plays a role, it might be directly related to the digestive system. In fact, it may be part of a vicious cycle. We have a problem in the gut that causes us to feel apathetic and not very good about ourselves. Then we don't fix the problem with proper nutrition and self care because we feel apathetic and

> If it keeps up, man will atrophy all his limbs but the push-button finger.
> - Frank Lloyd Wright

More than one billion people in the world are overweight.

Obesity is linked to metabolic syndrome, blood sugar and insulin disorders, heart disease, diabetes, hypertension, fatty liver, cancer, asth-ma, dementia, arthritis and kidney disease.

not very good about ourselves. It only spirals downward unless we recognize what is happening and make conscious choices that enhance our health and well being.

Motion and Emotion

In the chapter about children's imbalances—with our friends Winnie the Pooh, Tigger, and Eeyore—we discussed a little about the neurotransmitters (chemicals substances in the body that transmit messages to the brain) that are produced in the gut by the friendly bacteria. These neurotransmitters, like serotonin, GABA, and dopamine, affect your mood, your ability to concentrate, your quality of sleep, and more. If you are not getting proper neurotransmitters sent to your brain, it is very likely that you could be depressed. This could have you thinking twice about going to the gym, eating healthy, or even caring about what you look like. The real problem with adults is that they have been tolerating imbalance for so long, they just begin to accept this as feeling "normal." Imbalances begin to define our personalities and impact our lifestyle choices on a daily basis.

This apathy or indifference to doing what it takes to feel well develops into a cascade of symptoms and dis-ease. Remember the domino effect? Nearly all of the most common medical conditions facing adults and children can be seen as different stages of downed dominos. Nearly all of the dis-eases that develop start with the first domino falling down…usually related to your digestive system.

Again, instead of taking a pill to treat the symptoms, see a health care provider, such as a naturopath, who will help you consider why you are not digesting well. Are you absorbing the nutrients from your food? Even if you are eating nutritious foods, you become malnourished if you are not digesting properly and absorbing the nutrients. Undigested food sometimes sits in your body and putrefies and ferments, leading to gas, bloating, and toxins releasing into the body. These toxins stress the liver, which is responsible for cleansing and detoxing. This condition can lead to more serious problems, even if you are taking a drug to relieve you of your symptoms. Still, your liver is over-working to eliminate toxins from your body, making you more susceptible to toxins from the environment. And you are still malnourished.

New technologies, diagnostic software, and improved educational programs help health practitioners identify many underlying causes of disease. From a holistic view–taking into account your whole body and not just your digestive system–exercise and circulation are also an important part of your health story. Your body needs to be in motion, as in exercise, in order for your body to circulate and get rid of waste.

~✍

KNOW YOUR BODY

Let's get back to Humpty. His fall might have begun with a little light-headedness. Small symptoms often set off the domino effect, breaking down the system until it knocks us down completely. So don't ignore small signs. If you are always tired, have earaches, are frequently irritable, are occasionally light headed, have trouble concentrating, are troubled with achy muscles and joints, these may be symptoms or beginnings of larger issues.

Don't panic! Once you start eating healthier food, exercising, and making better choices about your health, your body will return to balance and harmony, and you will feel better both physically and emotionally. You will sleep better, feel more grounded, smile more, and be better prepared to celebrate life! The body has the amazing ability to heal itself if properly nourished.

~✍

DRUG WARNING

If you recall in chapter 2 with our friend Pig Pen, we talked about the micro-universe inside our digestive systems–the good bacteria and the intestinal bad guys, such as parasites, yeast, and fungi–and how imbalance causes the bad guys to thrive. The same thing happens when we use antibiotics. They wipe out both good and bad bacteria, but the troublemakers (the bad bacteria) come back quickly and upset the environment in of the internal world. Medical terminology refers to this as "dys-biosis," or the imbalance of life. Most dis-ease in the body begins when this imbalance occurs.

Also recall how the word "probiotic" means "for life" and "antibiotic" means "against life." The drug is not meant to harm you, but it is fighting to kill all bacteria instead of working to build a strong immune environment where healthy bacteria will thrive over bad. Again, let me stress that not all antibiotic use is bad, but we have definitely relied on them too much over the past years. I believe there is a correlation between this increased reliance and the dramatic rise of illnesses, both chronic and acute.

It's easy to have a doctor write a prescription and then do as we are told, but again, the message here is to be a conscious consumer. Modern health requires us to become more educated and make better choices for our health. We have been trained to trust in our doctors and even the government via the FDA (Food & Drug Administration). But do we trust too much without asking questions?

Science and technology have done wonders in many areas of healthcare, but too often we see drugs with serious side effects, including death, even after they have been through the FDA's safety procedures. The truth is, medicine is big business. The latest and greatest new pill is marketed to you, the consumer, to make lots of money for the company that makes it. The more drugs a person takes, the more profit the company makes. The system works better when there is imbalance, or dis-ease. That means that people need to be sick. I am not suggesting that all drugs are bad, by any means. But sometimes we need to question whether we really need to take that pill or at least we should understand what the drug does.

Drugs save lives all the time in emergency situations, such as heart attacks and other traumatic incidents. But perhaps we should consider options and alternatives when things are less serious. What did people do before pharmaceuticals? Actually, the drug companies haven't been around that long. People relied on natural substances, such as food, plants/herbs, water, and sun. Something as simple as the root or leaf of a plant can have powerful, healing effects. Several common drugs, which are now frequently prescribed, were originally created by studying the chemical structures and historic uses of plants. Learn about your health, your body, and your practitioner. Learn what you are taking and why, and remember to be a conscious healthcare consumer.

⊶

WHAT IS NATUROPATHIC MEDICINE?

Naturopathic Medicine is a unique system of healthcare, promoting natural healing and prevention of disease. A variety of non-invasive natural therapeutics and modalities are used holistically to treat both acute and chronic health conditions. Nutrition, lifestyle, and treating the whole person (mind, body, and spirt) are major areas of focus.

At this time, there are no strong federal guidelines making it clear to consumers what level of education a naturopath has completed. Professional training varies and may not be clear by the professional's title. In some states, naturopathic physicians are required to complete four years of training in clinical nutrition, acupuncture, homeopathic medicine, botanical medicine, psychology, and counseling (to encourage people to make lifestyle changes that support health). They graduate from an accredited, four–year graduate level naturopathic medical college program. In licensed states, a naturopathic physician (ND) with this level of education may be a primary care physician, having training hours that are comparable to an Allopathic practitioner (MD). However, some naturopaths receive degrees through a correspondence (distance-learning) program without having the benefit of hands-on clinical training/experience.

Currently, those who hold the titles of Doctors of Naturopathic Medicine, Doctors of Naturopathy, and Naturopathic Medical Doctor who have training in naturopathy and use both ND and NMD designations. Again, neither one gives any information about how extensive the training was in this specialized area. Stricter guidelines to distinguish types of practitioners, based on education levels, are now being considered in an effort to allow consumers to make educated choices when selecting health care providers.

A tip for conscious consumers: Ask questions! Ask about the duration, location, and depth of study. I am not saying that only the highest level of education is acceptable or that one kind of practitioner is good and another is bad. You will, undoubtedly, consider more factors than formal education–personal style, an ability to convey information, a sense that this is someone you can trust–to name a few. The important issue is that you have a right to know how much naturopathic schooling someone received, whether courses were in classrooms or online, and what kind of school was attended, so that you can make an informed choice based on standards that are important to you.

Regardless of which type of naturopath you choose, they all adhere to some basic philosophies of natural health and wellness.

6 Principles of Naturopathic Medicine

1   **First, Do No Harm** – Promote the use of safe, gentle, and natural therapies to improve well being while limiting risk and adverse effects.

2   **Healing Power of Nature** – Draw upon the body's innate healing intelligence. Nature guides and provides the knowledge used to bring the body into balance, moving towards a state of optimum health.

3   **Questioning for Causes** – Identify the source of dis-ease states, asking questions to find the causes, rather than just treating symptoms.

4   **Whole Person Treatment** – Assess the complex factors of human existence, including lifestyle, nutritional status, environmental toxins, emotional, mental, and spiritual health.

5   **Doctor as Teacher** – Educate patients with current, scientifically proven information and traditional origins of healing to promote self-responsibility for health and wellbeing. (The Latin root for "doctor" means "to teach.")

6   **Prevention** – Emphasize the significant benefits of healthy living practices in order to prevent the development of chronic illness and destructive disease states.

You are never too old to have a healthier ever after!

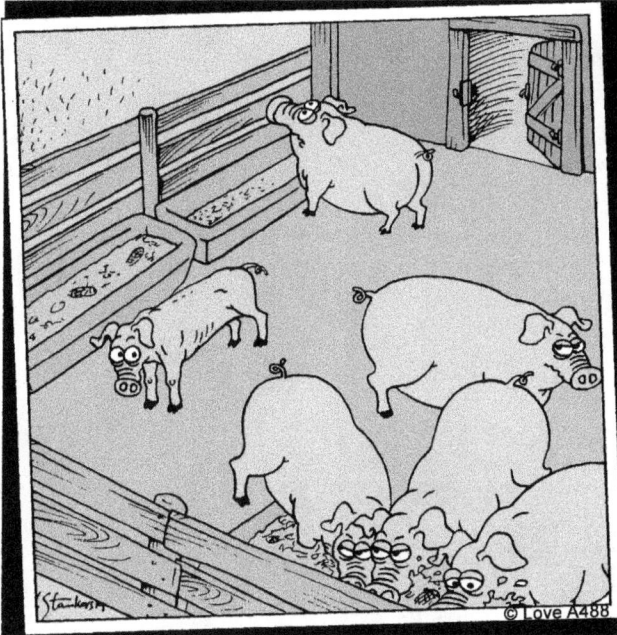

Although rejected by his peers, Slim continued to escape slaughter through diet and exercise.

CHAPTER 6

Mary Poppins
And Her Magical Medicine

Just a spoonful of sugar helps the medicine go down, the medicine go down, the medicine go down..."*

Who could forget the amazing Disney classic film nanny, Mary Poppins, who changed the lives of the Banks family? Mr. & Mrs. George Banks were very busy parents, something quite common in today's society, but they had the good fortune of having Mary Poppins land on their doorstep to take care of their children, Jane and Michael. Along with making sure their homework and chores were done each day (of course, with time for sunlight, fresh air, and laughter), as the song goes, Ms. Poppins also made certain that the children received a daily dose of "medicine."

❦

THE "MEDICINE"

Have you ever wondered what the "medicine" in the song actually was? A substance that tasted so bad, but was so important to give the children, that even a spoon full of sugar was acceptable in order to get it into their bodies? You might be surprised, but to solve this riddle you may have to think "outside the box" of what some consider a "medicine" today. The most likely answer to this question happens to be a natural remedy used for hundreds of years: fish oils– specifically, cod liver oil. Fish oils were popular in Europe as far back as the 17th century. A traditional medicinal drink in New Foundland, there was even a song written about this fishy elixir, touting some of its many health benefits.

Now a popular nutritional supplement, cod liver oil (as well as many other fish oils) has been extensively researched and found to support health. Cod liver oil is one of the best sources of Omega-3 fatty acids and contains high levels of essential fatty acids (EFAs), such as DHA (docosahexaenoic acid) and EPA (eicosapentaenoic acid). The body does not produce essential fatty acids, so we need to get them from our food, and studies show multiple health benefits when EPA and DHA are incorporated into the diet. Cod liver oil is also a healthy source of vitamins A and D, important for strong bones, proper liver function, good skin, and more. Fish and nuts are other good sources of EFAs. New and existing research continues to support the importance of good sources of fats in the diet. If you're concerned about the fat in healthy oils, be sure to read the Jack Sprat chapter!

---

*C*od Liver Oil

✧ Research shows that people who take cod liver oil every day have significantly less depression than those who don't.

✧ Cod liver oil has been shown to help stop cartilage breakdown due to arthritis.

✧ A large study showed an almost 25% reduced risk of breast cancer in women who used cod liver oil early in life.

So what about that spoon full of sugar you ask? Plain cod liver oil had a taste that's, well, a little difficult to swallow. However, the amount of sugar was small in comparison to the benefits of the oil, and people felt that the benefits of the cod liver oil far outweighed any negative effects of a little sugar. For many, the obstacle in taking this nutritional supplement was getting over the taste. Well, fear not my dear friends. New flavors of fish oil and cod liver oil are now available, including lemon, orange, mint, and peach. And for those who prefer to take a daily dose in pill form, fish oils are also available in capsules and gel caps. Most recommend taking your cod liver oil or other fish oils with meals, as the fats aid in the absorption of minerals in the food. If fish oil causes gas or discomfort, try taking a digestive enzyme with high levels of lipase. (More on enzymes in Chapter 8: Goldilocks)

෴

SOME MORE OF NATURE'S CURES

Nanny Poppins was not only giving the "medicine" and seeing that the chores were done, she knew the value of laughter and playtime. It's easy to forget in our busy lives just how curative it is to laugh and enjoy time outdoors.

Sunlight

The human body was designed to live in harmony with nature, and that meant some exposure to sunlight. Sunlight is good for our bodies, our moods, and even our sleep. Sunlight is so beneficial that some heath care practitioners use a treatment called heliotherapy, which uses the sun (helio) and its warmth, energy, and light as a therapeutic tool to treat illness or dis-ease. Exposure to sunlight should, of course, be in moderation.

> ## Vitamin D
>
> *Depending upon how often you are in the sun, you may want to adjust the amount of Vitamin D in your diet. You may need more in the way of a vitamin D supplement in late fall and winter, when outdoor exposure is limited compared to spring and summer seasons.*

Tanning beds can add a nice shade to your skin colors, but using light as a therapy usually covers a wider spectrum than those you will find in the neighborhood tanning salon. In 1903, the Nobel Prize for Medicine was given to Niels Ryberg Finsen for demonstrating that UV light was beneficial to patients with a variety of conditions, citing the importance of Vitamin D. The sun is a natural source of Vitamin D, which is important for strong bones and healthy bodies.

> Sources of vitamin D, such as cod liver oil, have been shown to reduce upper respiratory infections in children.

UV light, infrared saunas, and other resources to heliotherapy are becoming more popular. A good book to read more on this subject is *The Healing Sun: Sunlight and Health in the 21st Century* by Richard Hobday.

Vitamin A

Vitamin A is commonly known to be good for the liver and for eye health, but interestingly supplementation with Vitamin A often comes with a warning. High levels have reportedly been shown to be toxic to the liver, and women who are pregnant or nursing are usually told to limit intake. However, this does not mean that Vitamin A is bad for you. Many things that are otherwise beneficial are harmful at extremely high levels. In fact, Vitamin A found naturally in food–the way nature intended–is in a form the body can recognize and process, and is quite beneficial to your health.

Source: http://www.mercola.com

Laughter

They say "laughter is the best medicine," and it's true. One major way that laughter affects the body is through the immune system. Certain stress-related hormones that disrupt the immune system are reduced when we laugh. We also produce more disease fighting cells (called gamma-interferon t-cells). The physical moment of laughter even has subtle aerobic benefits, and it lowers blood pressure and increases oxygen intake.

Apparently, the body cannot tell the difference between laughter that is forced and laughter that comes naturally. Realizing this, people have begun to create "laughter clubs." Initiated in India, these clubs have now spread over most of the world. Even doctors are spreading the laughter, calling themselves "laughter coaches" who can teach you to laugh "effectively" so you can tee-hee your way to health, teaching people how

---

More of Nature's Simple Cures

In addition to laughter, other actions that increase endorphins and decrease blood pressure include prayer, meditation, and listening to music.

to laugh for the greatest health benefits. Laughter clubs usually get together in the morning for a bright, cheerful way to start the day.

Because laughter is a social phenomenon, the effects are strongest in a group. We also tend to laugh more within a group than we would alone. In fact, those who attend laughter clubs say that they begin by faking the laughs, but inevitably end up laughing genuinely because of all of the laughter around them. It's true that laughter is contagious!

Snapshots at jasonlove.com

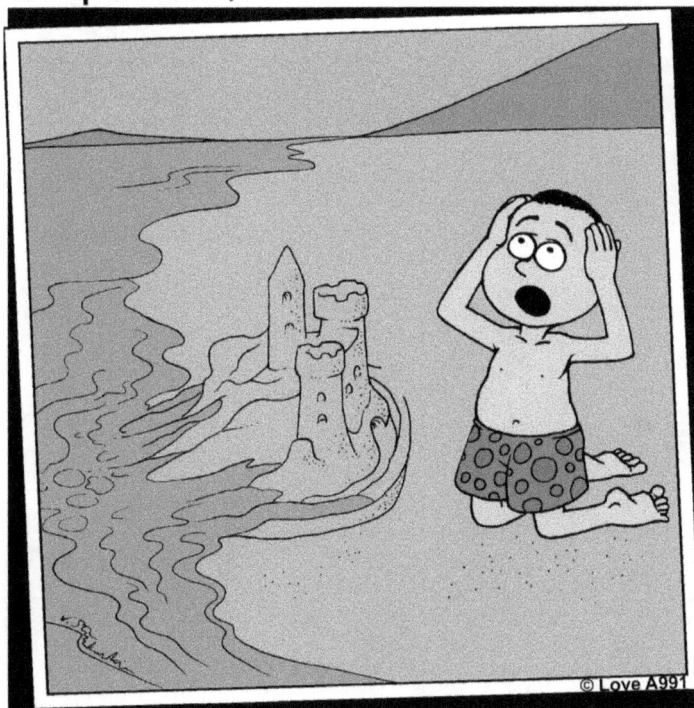

"No, cruel nature, WHY?"

CHAPTER 7

❦

Wile E. Coyote
Constant Cravings

*B*eep! Beep!"

There goes that darn Road Runner again. And we feel Mr. Wile E. (E for Ethelbert) Coyote's frustration over and over again as he tries to outwit and out-maneuver the blurred bird. But Road Runner gets away, and The Coyote is left splattered on the ground, only to get up, dust himself off, and go after the bird again.

Who better than The Coyote to look to as we examine cravings? His creator, Chuck Jones, based the character on a coyote in a Mark Twain story entitled "Roughing It"... Twain described his coyote as "a long, slim, sick and sorry-looking skeleton" and a "living, breathing allegory of Want." Wile E. most certainly had intense cravings, specifically for meat, more specifically for Road Runner. (He has The ACME Company delivering him all sorts of devices and weapons, but never does he order a pizza!)

❧

FOOD CRAVINGS

Food cravings are one way the body tells us what it needs in order to stay healthy. Before modern medicine and expensive diagnostic tests and equipment, we relied on signals the body gave us to help identify internal imbalances or deficiencies. We also had, long ago, an understanding that nature was providing, with each season, what was needed for health and survival. We still have, somewhere inside us, natural instincts.

> Lower glycemic foods (foods that don't significantly raise blood sugar) make you feel fuller than high glycemic foods (foods that dramatically raise blood sugar)

The flip side of cravings is that nutritional imbalances and chemical influences can lead us to crave things that are unhealthy. Many bad foods (and bad habits) are addictive, so how do we know when our cravings are instructive and when they are destructive? There is no easy answer. Common sense helps sometimes. Your body doesn't need anything in that powdered doughnut. But other times it is more confusing, and you will have to experiment to see what feels right for your body or see a health care practitioner to test your mineral and nutrient levels to see exactly what your body is lacking.

While some people crave sweets, some crave salt and others spicy food or bitter foods. Whether your cravings are for different tastes or flavors—even if they are for specific foods, such as chocolate or meat—if you can get a better understanding about the origins of these cravings, you can then keep them under control and improve your health at the same time.

Below are just a few explanations behind some common cravings:

Sugar

"I have a sweet tooth." "I just crave sugar." Sound familiar? Instead of viewing your cravings as a negative, consider that the body is trying to send you a message when you start to crave something sweet. If the body is low on an important nutrient, it is smart enough to send a message to your brain that it needs some more. Like any other craving, the craving for sweets may be your body trying to tell you something. Your body may be craving more glucose, or sugar, in the blood. Now you might be a little confused, because you know that today

> In experiments with rats, sugar can induce all of the effects of drug addiction: bingeing, withdrawal, cravings and cross sensitization.

we are eating more sugar and carbohydrates than our body needs, so how could we be low on glucose?

Remember, it's not always what you put in your body, but how your body reacts to what you consume. The stress of all the sugar causes an imbalance in blood sugar maintenance. The body works extra hard to keep glucose levels under control. But the body will continue its effort to maintain balance when under constant stress. It does its job of lowering the body's blood sugar to balance with the high sugar intake, and we end up with low blood sugar. We then crave more sugar and sweets. If we keep this cycle up, eventually the body cannot find balance and we end up with dangerous blood sugar levels.

Some people with sugar cravings, who feed them without checking in to see what's off balance in the body, develop Type 2 diabetes. Type 2 diabetes is a condition that develops over a period of time, the accumulation of dis-ease and imbalance resulting from mostly poor diet and lifestyle.

---

*C*oncerning Cravings

✦ Instead of simply fighting all of your cravings, examine where they come from and whether you are lacking something nutritionally. Consider working with a professional to identify deficiencies.

✦ If you choose to eat meat, consume small, reasonable quantities, and try to find free-range, hormone free meats.

Stress also factors in to diabetes and sugar cravings, affecting our ability to use sugar properly. When we consume sugary foods, the body, specifically the pancreas, produces insulin to help regulate blood sugar. (Insulin lowers blood sugar.) Cortisol, a hormone related to stress, is produced by the adrenal glands to stimulate insulin production, triggering a drop in blood glucose. So not only does improving your diet come in to play, but also better stress management impacts blood sugar control and diabetes. Consider what you eat, how much you eat, and even when you eat. Additionally, the overall health of your digestive system is vital. Yeast, bad bacteria, inflammation, and more can not only impair your ability to digest and absorb your food properly, but also may contribute through internal stress.

When craving sugar, realize also that refined sugar is an addictive substance for many. If you are a sugar-holic and simply cannot cut down, you might

> *Dieting increases food cravings, and fasting decreases them.*

want to try to cut it out completely for a while, along with refined carbohydrates (breads, chips, baked goods). Getting the sugars out of your system might get the cravings out of your system, too. Then you can put things back slowly and keep them in balance.

When considering your sugar intake, however, remember that all sugars are not the same. Avoid refined, processed, chemically bleached sugar and artificial sugar substitutes. The taste of sweet is not bad, but it should come from a natural source so that your body can process it effectively. An apple is sweet and has sugar, but that doesn't mean it is bad for you. Fruits and vegetables have natural sugars that the body utilizes in a healthy way. Raw, natural honey is great as well. Stevia (an herbal sweetener) is another good alternative to artificial sweeteners, as it comes from a natural source and is unprocessed. The more you eliminate the unnatural, processed sources of sweet in your diet, the more you will be able to taste the natural sugars found in food.

> *Beverages are not as filling as solid food, even if they are high in sugar, fat, or protein. Beverages that are all natural, fresh squeezed, and made from organic ingredients can still be very beneficial to your health.*

If you have sugar cravings, don't stress it! But try (ideally with a health care practitioner) to identify the reason your body is craving them and see what healthy habits you can develop.

Carbs

Complex carbohydrates are great, and many people don't even realize how many whole grains are available until they make a trip to the health food store. Brown rice is a healthy, whole grain that is common and easily available. Refined carbohydrates, such as white rice, breads, pastas, and baked goods, break down very quickly into sugars. If you are a carb or sugar addict, cutting down on one may only increase your consumption of the other. Many refined carbohydrates that we consume as snack food also have sugar and other unhealthy additives, such as partially hydrogenated oils. If you don't know what's in your favorite snack food, try reading the label. That way, even when you binge on your carbohydrates (as most of us do), you will at least be making a conscious choice about what you're putting in your body.

Salt

All matter, including the human body, is built on positive and negative charges. These charges are perhaps more familiar to us as electrolytes. Popular sports drinks have made this term a "buzz" word, but few people know what it means. The basic ingredients include salt, chloride, potassium and magnesium. In order for us to function properly, we need to maintain a balance of minerals in the body. Our kidneys and adrenal glands (little battery-like organs on top of the kidneys) help us manage stress, and need the positive and negative charges to keep us juiced up. When we are stressed, the minerals act as fuel to keep the batteries charged. Most people today are deficient in many of these minerals. We have numerous sources of stress. The food we eat has been depleted of these vital nutrients, and many foods we eat add to stress because they have been processed, overcooked, or filled with preservatives and chemicals. When we crave salt, we are often craving the minerals in unprocessed sea salt. Salt is a great source of minerals and our body instinctively knows that.

With that said, salt has

> ## SINGING THE PRAISES OF SEA SALT
>
> Throughout history, salt was actually considered to be a very valuable substance. Salt was often used as currency and many times was more treasured than gold. Soldiers were sometimes paid in salt for their service, early wars were fought over it, and it's even where the word "salary" comes from. All over the world, salt has played a role in economic, religious, social and political development. Salt also adds flavor to foods. Ask any decent chef!

been criticized for the past several years. High blood pressure has been connected by many in the medical community to the over consumption of salt. The increase in this dis-ease can most likely be shown to elevate around the same time we start processing and stripping all the minerals out of the natural sea salt. We also crave minerals and turn to salt when we feel stressed. But the problem is not the amazing natural substance, sea salt, but the kind of salt we have once it has been processed. When we turn to salty foods like chips and fried food, we are not even getting the minerals that may be causing the salt cravings, and the body has to work harder to digest these less-than-natural foods. This only adds to our stress by making our bodies work harder to digest these less than natural foods.

Some people just have an affinity for salt. The adrenal glands produce adrenaline and a hormone called cortisol, which is known as "the stress hormone," along with over 50 other essential body-regulating hormones. Adrenaline and cortisol are released under stress, pumping up the body to deal with an immediate physical threat. This response is known as "fight or flight." Few of our stresses today actually cause us to be ready to run or fight, but the body still reacts the same. If the body is pumping out too much stress hormone, it will be in a piqued state unnaturally, leading to chronic stress. You will also be overtaxing your adrenal glands, which can lead to fatigue, insomnia, and depression. Salt cravings may be one sign that your adrenals are fatigued and you are instinctively trying to build them back up.

RELAX—WITH SALT AND DARK CHOCOLATE!

When considering the underlying cause of hypertension or high blood pressure, we have to look at the stress hormone, cortisol. When you are under stress, the adrenal glands go to work and produce hormones, mainly cortisol. Cortisol has many effects on our body, including playing a role in blood sugar balance. Often, when we are stressed, we get constipated and/or our blood pressure rises. This is because cortisol is also vasoconstricting. Vasoconstriction is when blood vessels and other parts of the body "tighten up" or narrow. Interestingly, magnesium, an important mineral in which most people are deficient, is commonly found in both sea salt and dark chocolate, which relax muscles and cause blood vessels to open up, or vasodialate. Thus the new trend to add chocolate, specifically the dark variety, as a valuable "food group"!

The addition of some sea salt into your diet also helps rebuild the adrenal glands, so you may be instinctively self-medicating. Be conscious of when you are fatigued and notice whether some salt makes a difference. At the same time, be cautious of over-using salt and

> **T**IRED? Place a pinch of high mineral sea salt under your tongue when you're tired. Many notice an increase in energy.

be aware of your blood pressure. The best advice is always to work with a health care professional who is knowledgeable about nutrition. Treatment of adrenal fatigue involves relaxation, regularity of meals and bedtimes, healthy foods (whole grains, nuts and seeds, lots of veggies, high-quality oils such as flaxseed and olive oil), and a good dose of laughter now and then.

Sour

Most people don't worry about cravings for sour, and these cravings are less common than those for sugar or carbs. When we were young, many of us loved sour foods. In fact, the "Sour Patch Kids" candy is still one of the best selling treats on the market. Children will suck on lemons and many parents tell me that their child will suck on Vitamin C pills, ascorbic acid. As we get older, our taste buds become adulterated by all the sweets and sugar. But what could our bodies be telling us when we crave sour foods?

Many of the foods we eat are hard to digest and cause the body to become acidic. Sour foods are the taste our body knows to help us alkalize (become less acidic). Being too acidic and even too alkaline puts stress on the body, as the human system works in a constant effort to maintain balance, or homeostasis. A balanced PH, the scale to which acid and alkaline are measured, is quite significant

> **P**ICKLES AND ICE CREAM
>
> *Think about how strong cravings get when a woman is pregnant. The body's natural instincts are heightened in pregnancy; it makes sense that when this super-sensitive body is too acidic, it will have some pretty strong pickle cravings—though I'm not sure what drives the strawberry-ice-cream-in-the-middle-of-the-night craving!*

for optimal health. If your body craves for sour foods, perhaps you are too acidic. Again, these signals are meant to guide your dietary choices in a positive way. Nearly all sour foods are fermented; pickles, sour cream/kefir, sauerkraut, apple cider vinegar, etc.

Spicy

Some people love putting pepper or hot sauce on everything they eat. Unfortunately, these are often the same people who suffer from recurring heartburn or take antacids regularly. Heartburn and indigestion have several causes, including eating too quickly or too much, or having excessively hot food when our digestive systems don't have the strength to handle them. This weakness puts stress on the body when it tries to break down the food we eat and get proper nutrients from it.

According to Ayurvedic medicine (a 6,000+ year old "science of longevity" from India), this would be called weak agni. Our digestive systems have a fire, termed "Agni." This agni helps to transform the food we consume into useful nutrients our bodies can absorb. For many people in our society, this fire is dwindling or weak. Our digestive systems are struggling so the body calls for some outside "fire" support.

We have mentioned cortisol and stress many times in this section, but elevated cortisol is also thought to thin the lining of the digestive tract and halt production of important mucous that coats the walls of the system. This cycle may be why occurrences of ulcers, Irritable Bowel Syndrome (IBS), and even Crohns disease have been skyrocketing in our culture.

Unfortunately, the hot sauce and pepper (especially black pepper) seem to aggravate the continued inflammation and irritation of the lining of the digestive tract. Antacids and anti-inflammatory steroids seem to just cover up the problem, but do not resolve it. Instead of buying antacids in bulk, recognize the imbalance and the underlying cause of your symptoms. Eating more simple, easily digestible foods for a few weeks, incorporating some fermented foods into your diet, and supplementing with both digestive enzymes and probiotics (to produce more enzymes in the body) are great ways to address the underlying issues.

When replacing your processed table salt for unrefined, natural, mineral rich sea salt, also experiment by replacing your black pepper with cayenne or red pepper. Many find it less irritating and it can even help restore agni (the "fire" of your digestive system).

Cheese

Many of my clients say they crave cheese. My theory is that the body is still in search of more minerals; cheese is a good source of calcium, phosphorous, sodium, and more. Cheese may also be desired for those in need of good fats.

Meat

Many people do not consume meat, or any animal proteins/products, and the choice may be based on religious, personal, or health beliefs. For some though, the craving for meat is quite apparent. Like our friend Wile E., nothing can replace a good steak or piece of chicken.

Meat cravings can signal a number of deficiencies. Even if those deficiencies can be met without meat, the body knows that meat is a quick, easy way to get what is needed,

ENERGY DRINKS AND STIMULANTS

Everyone is searching for more energy. Nearly everyone suffers from not enough sleep, poor nutrition, and trying to cope with stressed out lives. So we turn to stimulants. Coffee has always been a staple, but over the past few years the "energy drink" category has exploded. Even though I look after my health, being a busy 30 something professional, I too experience moments where a little boost is helpful. When I look for a jolt of energy, I don't turn to high sugar sodas, and until recently, I have avoided the cans of liquid energy. So what if there are a few vitamins on the label? If the rest of the ingredients are unhealthy chemicals, artificial colorings, and preservatives, the product will be a stress on the body, and actually become a drain of energy in the long run.

Fortunately with new trends come new innovations. There are now energy drinks made using only natural ingredients. Yerba Mate is a plant with natural energy and antioxidants. Guarana is a plant being used more and more to replace synthetic caffeine in many products. Green tea is another natural source of energy.

Coffee is best when organic (so no pesticides or chemicals used on the coffee beans) and fair trade (supports the local farmers and agriculture who grow the beans). Also, I drink coffee black, or with little added ingredients. Coffee is natural. Artificial sweeteners, processed white sugar, chemically flavored "milk" and creamers are what really do the damage. There is now even vitamin fortified organic coffee on the market.

without waiting for the brain to look into it further and try different things. A craving wants what it wants (or in some cases needs)–in a hurry!

Deficiencies of iron, B vitamins (especially B12 and B6), and manganese (a trace mineral), zinc, or iron may result in meat cravings. Wile E. Coyote can choose to keep chasing Road Runner, but he may also want to learn which desert plants provide the missing nutrients. Clearly he's getting hungry by now. Maybe it's time to call for that pizza! But if he does want to fulfill his meat craving (and as a coyote he probably should), there are a few things he (and other meat eaters) should consider.

MEAT CHOICES

First, let me be clear that I am not advocating that everyone become a vegetarian. I am not vegan, vegetarian, raw, or any other label/classification. When people ask me, I tell then I am simply a conscious consumer. I make the best choices I can, based on the knowledge I have, combined with the situation at hand.

Meat Quantity: Excess animal protein and fat can be hard on our digestive systems. Our bodies use up great amounts of energy to break down and process the food we put in our mouths. Highly cooked animal proteins, when not broken down in our bodies properly, can actually start to rot, putrefy, and become toxic. If you eat meat, watch your portion size; colon care is central to good health and large portions of meat are hard to process. One book I recommend on the subject is, *A Guide to Better Bowel Care* by Bernard Jensen.

Meat Quality: Our increased consumption of meat and animal protein has put stress on both our internal, digestive environment and our external environment. The stress on the external environment causes conditions that further tax the internal environment of the body. The way animals are raised has been modified to keep up with the demand, from traditional farms to factory farms. The ugly conditions in which the animals are kept and the use of antibiotics and hormones to keep them alive longer to produce more and more, affect not only the health of the animal, but also the final product you bring home to your dinner table. If you choose to eat animal protein, look for quality sources; some are more natural and more humane than others. You can even have premium, high-quality meat delivered to your door, straight from the farm. (Try www.uswellnessmeats.com.)

The following are some general guidelines to consider if you choose to incorporate meat into your diet and lifestyle.

Look for:

- Organic, grass fed beef (Avoid very well done meat. The less cooked the better; at least try medium or medium rare)
- Free range chicken and eggs (preferably with high omega-3)
- Wild fish or line caught (instead of farm raised)

❧

OTHER COMMON CRAVINGS

Cigarettes, alcohol, drugs, and even sex:

When do most people crave or turn to these? Usually when dealing with stress, either acute or chronic. Even after sex (a good stress), people are known to smoke a cigarette as the adrenal glands are looking for replenishment. Yes, your adrenal glands also produce your sex hormones, so the rush you just enjoyed called upon those glands to be recharged. Hard day at work? Alcohol is a relaxant, similar to the mineral, magnesium, almost always deficient and what our bodies are craving. Sleep meds and anti-anxiety pills are just pharmaceutical patches for underlying nutritional imbalances.

Try eating more fresh fruits and vegetables, getting quality minerals and foundational nutritional support from good dietary supplements, while developing other stress management techniques, such as increased exercise, yoga, breathing, and meditation. I am in no way suggesting giving up the occasional and responsible drink of alcohol, becoming abstinent or not taking a pharmaceutical drug when necessary. I am simply suggesting that we can become less dependant on the substances we crave by strengthening and nourishing our bodies.

Manifest plainness, Embrace simplicity, Reduce selfishness,
Have few desires. - Lao-tzu

CHAPTER 8

———— ·//· ————

Goldilocks
And the Carb Crash

U*m-mmm! It was just right, and so she ate and ate and ate until there was not a bit of porridge left in the Baby Bear's little bowl… Goldilocks tried the littlest bed, and it was just right, and so she curled up and was soon fast asleep.*

Poor Goldilocks went for a hike and forgot to take any trail mix, snacks, or energy/protein bars. After a few hours, she felt her blood sugar getting a little low, and her stomach started to rumble. Knowing the importance of eating small, frequent meals to maintain proper blood sugar, she started looking around the woods for something she could eat. Then Goldilocks spied a house in the forest and decided to see if she could ask the occupants for a snack. She knocked on the door, and to her surprise, the door creaked open. Now maybe it was the low blood sugar affecting her better judgment, but she decided to go inside the house.

Once inside, Goldilocks noticed three bowls of porridge on the table. If you don't know porridge, perhaps you are familiar with grits, oatmeal, farina—or even consider a big bowl of pasta. She sits down, and although she chooses the smallest of the three bowls, she is still smaller than a small bear and what felt "just right" was still probably a bit too much. She becomes sleepy and has to lie down for a nap. Goldilocks got "carb coma."

ಿ∾9)

When you eat foods like porridge or pasta or donuts, your body has to digest them with its own enzymes, this increases the energy demand in the digestive system and reduces the available energy to other systems of the body. It is a supreme waste of resources and metabolic energy. Goldilocks wasn't lazy; she was just digesting her food the hard way.

Outside of fairy tales, bears are much smarter eating things like sushi, fresh berries and grubs, and of course the occasional little blonde intruder (kidding). Diets rich in enzymes bring robust health, and no sudden napping at inopportune times.

What are enzymes, anyway? (You ask all the right questions!) Enzymes are essential protein units that sustain all life. Enzymes play a role in every move you make, breath you take, action, reaction, etc.

Enzymes, tiny elements of energy, can be affected by many things, including temperature. Enzymatic reactions speed up as temperature increases, and slow down when temperature decreases. Seems simple enough, right? Here's the catch. Above a certain temperature, enzymes stop speeding up–they pretty much explode. The scientific term is "denature." Today most food is cooked, processed, microwaved, or somehow manipulated in a way that the enzymes are destroyed or made less effective. This goes directly against the way Nature had intended the food to be consumed, and therefore the body has to react in an effort to accommodate. Most often, this involves using up valuable energy and enzymes produced by the body.

ಿ∾9)

People who live on cooked, refined, or processed foods create a high demand for digestive enzymes which will often result in an enzyme deficiency pretty quickly and can, if left unchecked, contract one of today's common conditions such as indigestion, heartburn, or acid reflux. Depleted enzyme stores also contribute to type 2 diabetes and obesity. When you have food in your stomach, energy is diverted towards digestion, and enzymes are called to do the work. When you don't have enough enzymes, your body stops functioning optimally, and you start looking for the TV Guide. To avoid the coma, choose foods that are rich in enzymes such as raw fruits and vegetables, non-pasteurized dairy, fermented foods, sushi, and salads.

Dr. Edward Howell, an authority on enzyme science said, "The length of one's life is held to be inversely proportional to the rate of energy expenditure." It sounds like something you forgot from geometry, but Howell is right: the faster we burn our enzymes, the sooner we reach the end of this whole life thing. His argument applies to every creature of the forest. They may not understand science, but they instinctively know how to manage their enzymes.

The *Pottenger Cat Study* 2 and other related work have shown that for animals in captivity, mortality rates are highest when the creatures are fed enzyme-poor, "dead" foods such as white bread, boiled potatoes, and cooked meat. (Sounds similar to the Standard American Diet, doesn't it?) Not only are their life spans cut short, but they also stop reproducing.

In recent years, zoos and pet stores have modified their fare to include raw, living foods such as fresh fruits and vegetables and even raw meat. As chance would have it, the animals have responded in kind. They are living longer, showing fewer signs of illness, and reproducing (even in captivity). Let this be proof that a simple change of diet can do wonders for your mojo.

In the book, *Everything You Need to Know About Enzymes* the author, Tom Bohager, recommends three simple steps to improving your health:

1. Eat more raw foods. Incorporate one raw food meal per day. Having a salad for lunch instead of a hamburger will spare your enzymes and even give you more energy for the afternoon.
2. Eat fewer total calories per day. Studies have shown that eating less per day can add years to your life.

---

2 The *Pottenger Cat Study* is a ten-year nutrition study on approximately 900 cats, covering three generations. Designed to mirror Dr. Weston A. Price's human findings of health and nutrition relationships in traditional cultures, the study found that a diet of raw meat and dairy proved significantly better than a diet of cooked meat and pasteurized/ evaporated milk. Degenerative diseases, diminished energy, shortened life-span, and inability to reproduce were all observed in the group fed cooked meat and modified dairy.

ENZYMES	DIGESTIVE	THERAPEUTIC
Alpha galactosidase	Breaks down carbohydrates, such as raffinose stacchyose. Helps digest raw vegetables and beans	Reduces gas and bloating
Amylase	Breaks down carbohydrates starch, glycogen, and polysaccharides	Assists in balancing histamine levels, helps with allergies, reduces food cravings, and increase blood sugar
Beta Glucanase	Breaks down beta D-glucan components associated with grains such as barley, oats and wheat	Helps with malabsorption, and may be beneficial for food and environmental allergies, gas, and bloating
Bromelain	Breaks down protein	Breaks down protein, and reduces inflammation
Catalase		Antioxidant that breaks down hydrogen peroxide into water
Cellulase	Breaks down cellulose, and helps to release nutrients in both fruits and vegetables	Breaks down chitin, a cellulose like fiber found in the cell wall of candida
DPP IV Protease	Breaks down gluten and casein peptide	
Glucoamylase	Breaks down carbohydrates, and polysaccharides into glucose	Assists in balancing histamine levels
Hemicellulase	Breaks down carbohydrates and polysaccharides found in plant foods	
Invertase	Breaks down carbohydrates, especially sucrose	
Lactase	Breaks down milk sugar	Helps with lactose intolerance
Lipase	Breaks down lipids and improves fat utilization	Supports gallbladder function, helps with cholesterol, skin issues, hormones, vertigo, diabetes, and helps to break down Essential Fatty Acids (EFA's).

Maltase	Breaks down carbohydrates, malts and grain sugars, and complex and simple sugars	
Mucolase		Breaks down mucous, and helps with congestion and sinus infection
Nattokinase		Breaks down fibrin, and assists with blood clots, circulation, and cardiovascular support
Papain	Breaks down protein, and soothes G.I. tract	Breaks down protein and reduces inflammation
Pectinase	Breaks down carbohydrates and pectin found in fruits and vegetables	Helps with mineral absorption
Phytase	Breaks down carbohydrates and phytic acid found in the leaves of plants	Helps with mineral absorption
Protease	Breaks down protein	Bonds with alpha 2-macroglobulin to support immune function, reduces inflammation, and increases circulation
Serratiopepti-dase		Breaks down fibrin, mucous, and reduces inflammation
Xylanase	A type of Hemmicellulase found in grains that breaks down soluble fiber	

3. Take enzymes in the form of a dietary supplement whenever you eat, whether the meal is small or large, cooked or raw.

Taking an enzyme supplement is helpful when suffering from digestive issues, but also spares your own enzyme resources. Additionally, it lets you enjoy the freedom of enjoying some foods that may be harder to process on your own–maybe a steak or a slice of pizza. Whatever your dietary choices, your body will appreciate the extra enzymes–and you will quickly feel the difference.

❧

Learning about and appreciating the role that enzymes play allows us to make better choices about what we eat, making an effort to look for the choices that assist the body in digestion and avoid those that drain energy and enzyme stores. Even when we are watching what we eat, our busy schedules have us often eating out in restaurants, airports, or at work. Fresh, nutritious food is not always available, or perhaps not what we choose to eat at that moment. That's okay. The more frequently we make good choices when available, the less impact those occasions have on our overall health.

Understanding the importance of enzymes is just another way we can make better choices and continue down the path to a healthier ever after.

While most of this chapter has focused on taking enzymes with food to aid in digestion, enzymes have also been shown to have significant health benefits when taken on an empty stomach. Enzymes taken on an empty stomach have been shown to reduce inflammation, support the immune system, help with sugar cravings, treat allergic symptoms, and much more. The best thing about enzymes is that they are safe, natural, and have very few contra-indications (especially plant-based, vegetarian enzymes).

In the early 1900's, Dr. John Beard wrote a paper entitled, " The Enzyme Treatment of Cancer and its Scientific Basis." This work, greatly ridiculed at the time, was written to promote enzyme therapy as a method of cancer treatment. After all these years, the treatment is gaining acceptance and enzymes are often used, in concert with other methods, for treating cancer. Enzymes are also used to treat numerous other conditions.

Proteolytic enzymes can be taken on an empty stomach both as a preventative, and in larger doses, to help support the immune system in times of illness. Protease is the enzyme responsible for breaking down proteins. Major athletic programs use this enzyme to reduce swelling, inflammation, and to shorten recovery time after sports injuries.

Dis-Ease

You may have noticed that, throughout this book, the word disease is usually hyphenated. This is done with intent in an effort to emphasize the loss of balance, comfort, stability, etc. in a person's body and/or life. Health is not the absence of every symptom or some unrealistic, super-human state of health. Health is a range in which the body is somewhat balanced and in a relatively comfortable state of being, a state of ease. When the state of ease and health is compromised, we suffer with dis-ease. Minor dis-ease feels manageable. We can often make a change and see some result. When we're dealing with more serious dis-eases, we need more patience, care, and time to bring our bodies back to a healthy state of balance and ease.

White blood cells are your body's defense against infection. An increase of white blood cells in your lab work shows not only that you have an infection, but also that your body is working to fight it. Think of white blood cells as ambulances, rushing out to the scene of injury in your body. Now think of enzymes as the emergency medical personnel who ride in the ambulances to the site of the injury/accident. Just having more ambulances won't help you if you don't have enough personnel/enzymes to do the work of care and healing. You need to have enough personnel–protease enzymes–to help your immune system regain its strength.

Amylase enzymes, the ones that break down sugars, have been shown to reduce histamine response, reducing symptoms related to allergies. Taking amylase away from food has also been said to help control sugar cravings.

Breaking down fat requires lipase enzymes. Some suggest that nearly all people who are classified as obese are deficient in lipase. Taking enzymes may help support weight loss/management, and supplementation may help take stress off the gallbladder and liver.

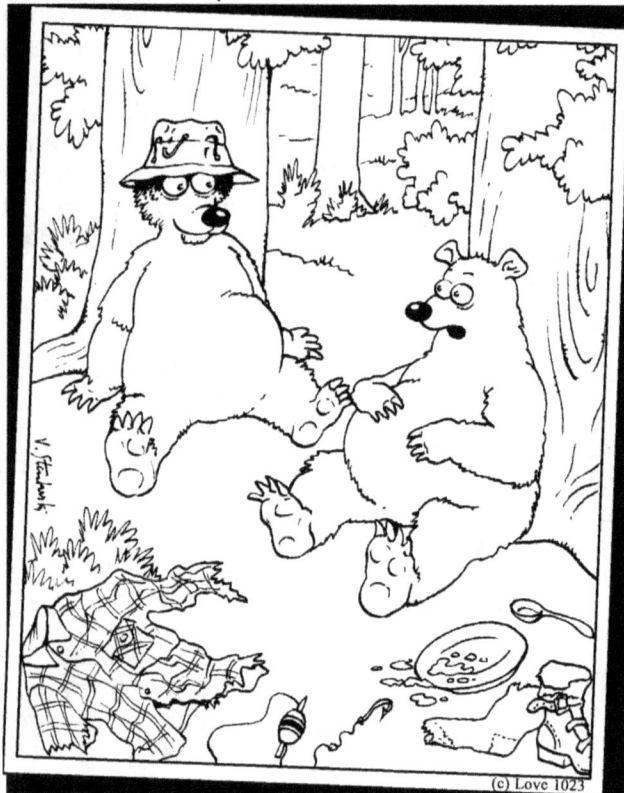

"I shouldn't have gone back for seconds,
but I've got a weakness for vegetarians."

Notes

CHAPTER 9

❧

Little Miss Muffet
Yes, Whey!

Little Miss Muffet, sat on a tuffet (a little stool or chair), eating her curds and whey. Along came a spider, sat down beside her, and said, "Hey, what's in the bowl @&%!#?"

—The Little Miss Muffet story as retold by comedian Andrew Dice Clay

While this version is not the most eloquent of poetry, the question raised by the spider is a pretty basic one. What is whey? Many protein shakes and bars list some form of whey protein on the label. Where does whey come from? What is its nutritional value? Was "little" Miss Muffet trying to bulk up?

❧

WHY WHEY?

When a glass of milk is allowed to sit out in room temperature for a while, a noticeable separation occurs. Now you might already be thinking, who lets milk sit out on the counter? Keep in mind that the invention of the modern refrigerator is roughly a hundred years old, and the use of domesticated animal milk goes back over 8,000 years (Even the tale of Ms. Muffet goes back to 1805). Sometimes this separation occurs naturally, while enzymes can speed up the process. One half of this equation is the curds.

You don't see any protein bars with "curds" on the label, but like whey, curds are also a type of protein, called casein. The casein part of milk is most often used to make cheese. Curds are where most of the protein comes from in cottage cheese, a "dieter's" staple. Casein protein, for some, is hard to digest. The liquid part that remains, called whey, provides a valuable source of digestible protein, along with other important nutrients. Miss Muffet may not have known this, but whey protein has been shown to build and repair muscle, be a valuable tool in weight maintenance, provide a healthy source of energy, and even support a healthy immune system.

Most people are probably familiar with protein powders for body building and bulking up, but the truth is, Little Miss Muffet wasn't trying to be "Big" Miss Muffet. High-quality proteins are important for people of all ages. Then again, not all protein powders are created equal. Whey protein is said to have high amounts of amino acids, the building blocks of protein, helping to build, repair, and heal muscle tissue. Other types of protein powders are now available in the health industry as well: hemp, rice, pea, and, of course, soy protein. Some people choose non-dairy alternatives because they do not want to eat animal-derived products and prefer plant sources, but many avoid whey protein because they are lactose intolerant, and have had issues digesting whey protein in the past.

A brief Note on Soy and Soy Protein

Of course, this preference for processing is not limited to just animal-based products. The recent explosion of soy products should raise some flags of caution. The processing that goes into soy protein isolate and textured soy protein products may yield unhealthy and potentially dangerous byproducts. Soy contains phytic acid, a substance not meant to be consumed in large amounts. It blocks the assimilation of important nutrients such as calcium, magnesium, zinc, and others. Soy also contains trypsin inhibitors, substances that interfere with the absorption of protein. If you are going to incorporate soy into your diet, I recommend soy foods that have been naturally fermented: miso, tempeh, and natto.

Source: www.westonaprice.org

൭

WHEY-ING THE OPTIONS

While whey can be very beneficial, not all whey is the same, and understanding the differences is important to making good product choices.

Liquid Form

Whey in liquid form is a natural product, occurring from the separation of milk. Liquid whey protein contains important immune-supporting components including lactoferrin, lactoglobulin, and IgG. Whey also contains other nutrients found in dairy, such as some casein protein, fat, cholesterol, and lactose. Whey, when in liquid form, can be used to soak flour before baking and grains before cooking to improve digestibility. Before you go to bed, use whey to soak your oats overnight. Wake up and prepare them the way you normally do. The oats will taste the same, but your body will know the difference. (For more information, I recommend that you read *Nourishing Traditions*, by Sally Fallon.)

> Unlike drinks with fructose or glucose, whey protein drinks do not raise blood sugar, stimulate insulin, or increase hunger.

Powder Forms

Whey Protein Concentrate

Whey contains more than just whey protein, and some of the other components may make it challenging to digest the protein in powder form. As a result, the manufacturers decided to first reduce the amount of fat, lactose, casein, and other ingredients. This leaves a higher percentage, or increased concentration of the whey protein in the powder. This is known as whey protein concentrate. Generally, whey protein concentrate is a decent product, but when you are looking for health benefits specifically from whey protein, it may be better to select whey protein isolate (which is often easier to

> Whey protein boosts the immune system.

digest).

Whey Protein Isolate

> **W**hey protein is antimicrobial.

Whey protein isolate means that the whey has been isolated; most other ingredients have not just been reduced, but pretty much eliminated from the powder, leaving just the whey protein–hopefully still in a digestible form with the immune benefits intact. Whey protein isolate comes in three forms. The healthiest, most natural form is ultra-filtered, or micro-filtered. But, being a conscious consumer, you'll want to read about all three!

1. *Hydrolyzed Whey Protein Isolate:* This process separates the whey protein in a way that is not very natural. In fact, the proteins are chopped up by enzymes and temperature, changing their original structure, often making them hard to digest. Hydrolyzing proteins may also produce an unhealthy byproduct, monosodium glutamate, more commonly known as MSG.

2. *Ion Exchange:* This is a fairly popular process, as nearly all of the other ingredients are stripped away, leaving a high percentage of whey protein. Unfortunately, the process uses chemicals such as sodium hydroxide and hydrochloric acid, destroying some of the proteins in the process. In addition to not being a very natural process, nearly all of the valuable immune properties found in whey protein are also stripped out, along with

> **N**OURISHING TRADITIONS
>
> *To find out more about whey, look for a favorite book of mine called **"NOURISHING TRADITIONS"** by Sally Fallon. It's a great cookbook, and unbelievable nutrition guide as well!*

the lactose, fat, and other ingredients. You may be getting protein, but you are missing out on the immune benefits of whey protein.

3. *Ultra-Filtered/Micro-Filtered:* This method utilizes screens, filters, and natural membranes to separate the whey protein by particle size and weight, without the use of chemicals or high temperatures. This simple approach may cost a little more, but you get a very

digestible, absorbable protein, isolated from nearly all of the other ingredients, while still containing those important immune-supporting elements. This is the most natural approach to isolating whey protein ,and the form I recommend.

As you can see, not all whey proteins are created equal. On the surface, they have the same name and may appear to be similar, but in reality, some are manipulated and transformed so far from what nature intended that this once healthy substance becomes unhealthy. This is often the case–from raw milk being converted to an enzyme-deficient, pasteurized, homogenized liquid; to healthy oils being transformed into toxic, hydrogenated fats; and to whey protein being potentially manipulated into MSG or non-digestible protein powders.

*W*hey protein is an antioxidant.

Learning about the origins of and processes behind producing our foods is essential for health. Proteins derived from animals, whether in powder form or a steak, have the potential for containing antibiotics, hormones, toxic residues, etc. Plant-based foods and supplements can also be tainted with chemicals and other unhealthy substances. This is why, even though buying foods and products from reputable health food stores may be a little more expensive, it's a worthwhile investment. Most stores that are part of the natural food and products industry make an effort to only offer foods and products free of unhealthy hormones, antibiotics, chemicals, etc. They hire people to investigate the ingredients in a product, hoping to provide you, the consumer, with a product that will have more benefits than drawbacks. Shopping in health food stores is a good way to help you make the right choice; they are there to help you be a conscious consumer.

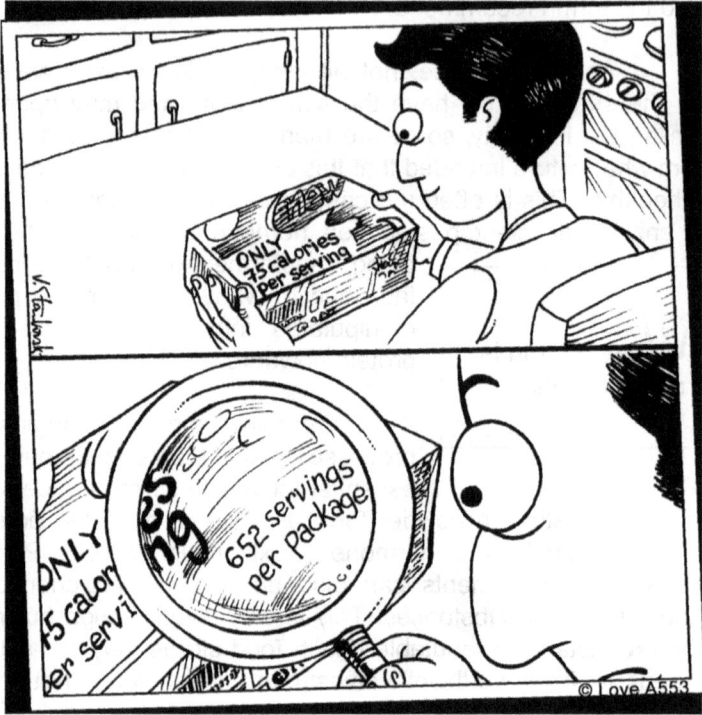

Notes

CHAPTER 10

Jack Sprat
Needed Some Fat

"Happiness is not a matter of intensity but of balance and order and rhythm and harmony." - Thomas Merton

Original Version: *"Jack Sprat could eat no fat, his wife could eat no lean. And so betwixt the two of them, they licked the platter clean."*

A Modern-Day Version: *"Jack Sprat ate no fat, his wife ate no lean, but both were eating wrong–they were way too extreme!"*

Although I applaud the idea of sharing a meal as a way of eating smaller portions and reducing caloric intake (a good idea in general), neither an all-fat or a completely no-fat diet is the best approach to dealing with weight loss and healthful eating. We have all heard the saying, "everything in moderation." It's a lesson I learned from my grandparents. This is good advice for all of us, including Mr. And Mrs. Sprat. Some fats are harmful and should be avoided, but others are essential for good health.

The subject of fats raises many questions. What are the good fats, and how should they be consumed? Which fats are unhealthy, and how can they be avoided? Shouldn't I be choosing products labeled "fat free"? Let's start by clearing some fat-free confusion. "Fat-free" products may cost you more because what replaces the fat is usually less health-ful than the fat itself. In fact, on fat free fad diets, many people actually gain weight more than they lose because they eat so much more as a result of not feeling satisfied.

A simple rule for knowing which fats to eat is to stick with the most

SNACK TIP

Grind up some hemp and flaxseeds into a shake or sprinkle on a salad.

natural forms, those with the least amount of processing or man-made influence. Avoid or minimize unhealthy fats, such as margarine, trans-fat, shortening, vegetable oils, soy, corn, canola oils, and those described as "hydrogenated" or "partially hydrogenated." Moderately consume good fats such as avocado, butter (organic, raw is best), coconut oil*, olive oil, palm oil*, flaxseed oil, omega 3 rich oil, cod liver oil, and ghee*(clarified butter). * Good for frying.

Some of the good fats/oils are great for cooking, such as ghee (clarified butter, used for many years in India), and coconut oil, which is organic and unrefined. Other fats/oils make good salad dressings and marinades, such as extra virgin olive oil. Others are best taken as supplements from the health food store, including cod liver oil, flax oil, fish oils, and evening primrose oil. Incorporate a variety of healthy fats into your diet, in moderate amounts. Branch out and try different oils on salads or drizzled over steamed vegetables. You will not only enjoy the different tastes, but they offer a variety of health benefits as well.

Sometimes we become so focused on quantity that we forget about quality. Imagine, for example, two "healthy" energy bars. You decide to watch your weight and are looking for more healthful snacks. Bar #1 has 5

Essential Fatty Acids must be eaten, since the body cannot make these good fats and cannot function properly without them.

More than half of the dry weight of the brain consists of good fats.

Omega 3 oils improve cholesterol, reduce risk of heart disease, strengthen hair, help manage diabetes, and do so much more.

Good fats can prevent irregular heart rhythms.

EPA, a good fat, lowers cholesterol and prevents heart attacks.

grams of fat and bar #2 has 9 grams of fat. That's nearly twice as much. Your first instinct may be to go for the one with fewer total grams of fat, but like any good conscious consumer, you take a look at the ingredient list. Although bar #1 has a lower total fat content, it contains low quality and hydrogenated, processed oils. Trans

> *If olive oil comes from olives, where does baby oil come from?*

fats are now banned from use in many products and even barred from use in New York restaurants because they have been shown to cause heart disease and other serious health risks. Now, upon inspection, you realize that the 9 grams of fat found in bar #2 are from organic nuts, seeds, and cold-pressed coconut oil. These are healthy sources of fat that the body can recognize and utilize effectively. Fat from almond butter, avocados, flaxseeds, etc. is actually beneficial, while the types of fat found in fast food, doughnuts, and fried chicken are harmful.

Some key words to look for in identifying good, healthy fats:

- Organic
- Cold pressed (no heat used in the process)
- Extra virgin
- Omega 3
- Unrefined
- DHA and EPA

> *Why do "fat chance" and "slim chance" mean the same thing?*

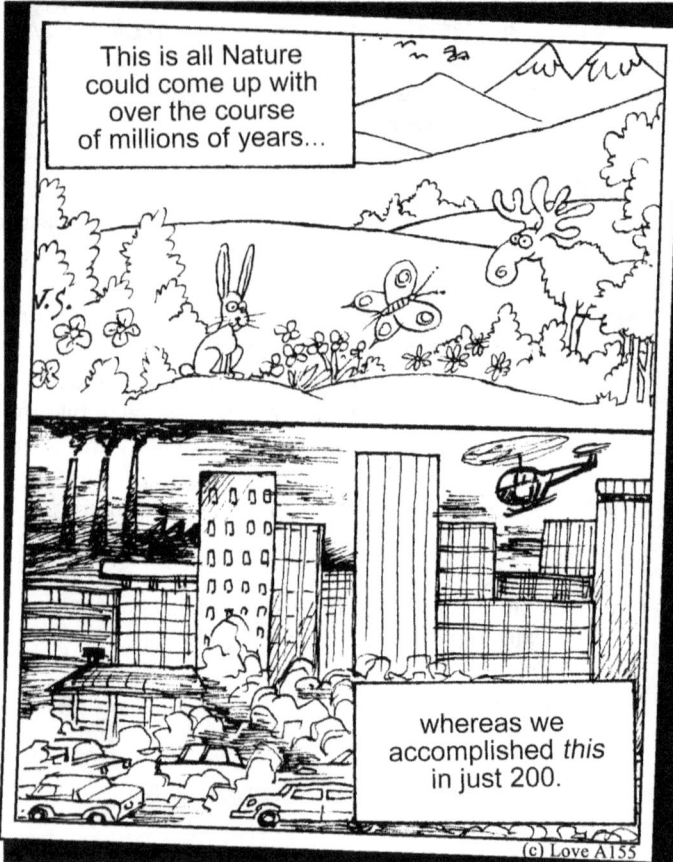

Notes

CHAPTER 11

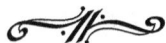

Jack and Jill
The Water Tumblers

Original Version: *"Jack and Jill went up the hill to fetch a pail of water."*

A Modern-Day Version: *"Jack and Jill went to the store to buy some bottled water."*

Back in the days of Jack and Jill, water safety meant "Look where you're going when you come down that hill," today, water safety is much more complex. Falling down a hill is the least of our concerns!

❧

WATER QUALITY

So how does a conscious consumer look at water? We are constantly seeing words and terms spring up, like filtered, mineral, flat, sparkling, carbonated, vitamin-infused, glacial, pure, reverse osmosis, etc. Some water is called "hard" and other "soft," relating to the amount of minerals that are dissolved in the water. Soft water is said to be easier on the plumbing in your home, but maybe it's harder on the plumbing in your body. Should you drink sparkling or flat? Mineral water or distilled? Are plastic bottles a concern? How would you navigate the waves of new water filters and bottled waters to select the right ones? We are awash in water options and confusion. Unfortunately, the days are gone when we simply turned on the tap and trusted that we had good, safe water.

Research has linked chlorine in both bathing and

TYPES OF WATER	DEFINITION	CONTAMINANTS REMOVED
FILTERED	This is a type of drinking water that has been treated with processed such as, a layer of GAC (granulated activated charcoal) or sand, reverse osmosis or distillation, to remove bacteria and dissolved solids.	Contaninants Removed
TYPES OF FILTERED WATER GAC (granulated activated charcoal)	GAC (granulated activated charcoal), also called **activated charcoal** or **activated coal**. Activated charcoal is good at trapping other carbon-based impurities ("organic" chemicals), as well as things like chlorine. Many other chemicals are not attracted to carbon at all -- sodium, nitrates, etc. -- so they pass right through. This means that an activated charcoal filter will remove certain impurities while ignoring others. It also means that, once all of the bonding sites are filled, an activated charcoal filter stops working. At that point, you must replace the filter.	Chlorine,Cysts, Suspended solids, Protozoa,Organic chemicals, Arsenic, Lead, VOC's, Total Trihalomethanes (TTHM)
DISTILLED Steam Action	Distilled water is water that has virtually all of its impurities removed through distillation, which involves boiling & condensing the steam into a clean container.	Chlorine, heavy metals, organic and inorganic chemicals, micro organisms, **Fluoride**, Total Dissolved Solids (TDS), Asbestos
REVERSE OSMOSIS GAC, Membrane	Reverse osmosis uses a membrane type for filtration that is semi-permeable, allowing pure water to pass through it, while rejecting the contaminants that are too large to pass through the tiny pores in the membrane. A typical RO system is composed of an array of granular activated carbon (GAC) pre-filters, the reverse osmosis membrane, storage tank.	Chlorine, heavy metals, organic, and inorganic chemicals, micro organisms, **Fluoride**, Total Dissolved Solids (TDS), Total Trihalomethanes (TTHM)
KANGEN-ALKALINE-IONIZED COMBINED GAC (granulated activated carbon), and Electrolysis	There are two ways the quality of kangen or alkaline water are measured - by how acid or alkaline the water becomes (pH), and by how much ionization occurs (ORP). The word "KANGEN" scientifically means reducing or deoxidizing. It also means back to origin, "renewal" and that is what it does, restoring your body back to a balanced state. They adopted a name "kangen" that is used to describe healthy, clean, alkaline water that has no impurities and is ionized. It allows your body to absorb all nutrients much faster. First, the water is purified when it passes through the solid carbon block filter. Next, the water is ionized through electrolysis, as it passes through seven platinum-coated titanium plates. The electrolysis process splits the water into two parts: alkaline (hydrogen-rich) and acidic (oxygen rich). The resulting alkaline water, or Kangen water, has incredible deoxidizing properties.	Chlorine, Cysts, Suspended solids, Protozoa, Onorganic, and Inorganic chemicals, Arsenic, Lead, Voc's, Total Trihalomethanes (TTHM)

MINERAL	Mineral water comes from a natural well or spring. Mineral H20 contains no less that 250 PPM total dissolved solids.	Total Solids (TDS) are primarily minerals/salts, but can also include organic matter
SPARKLING	Sparkling Water - the fizzy kind? What makes the fizz? This H20 contains the same amount of "carbon dioxide" that it had when it emerged from its source.	Carbonated water, also known as sparkling water, is plain water into which carbon dioxide gas has been dissolved
GLACIER/ ARTESIAN	Artesian water comes from a source deep within the earth, protected by layers of clay and rock. There is no opening to the surface. As a result, the water never comes in contact with the air, from environmental pollutants and containments.	Mineral, metal, Compounds, and salts are very low. Oxidization
HARD WATER	Hard water is water that contains calcium and magnesium salts dissolved in it. These salts make it difficult to get soap to lather, can leave deposits on clothes that were washed in hard water, and can also leave deposits in water pipes. Hard water is not harmful for drinking.	High Mineral Content Calcium, Magnesium Salts
SOFT WATER	Soft water does not contain these salts, and the problems associated with hard water are not present. Soft water reduces the surface tension, allowing for better suding and lathering of soaps. Water softeners run hard water through a filtration system to remove the calcium and magnesium salts from the water to change it from hard to soft.	Soft water is the term given to describe types of water that contain few or no calcium or magnesium ions.

Essential Water

❖ Our bodies are made up of about 80% water.

❖ The planet is covered nearly 2/3rds by water.

❖ The weight you lose directly after working out or playing an intense sport is from water loss, not fat loss.

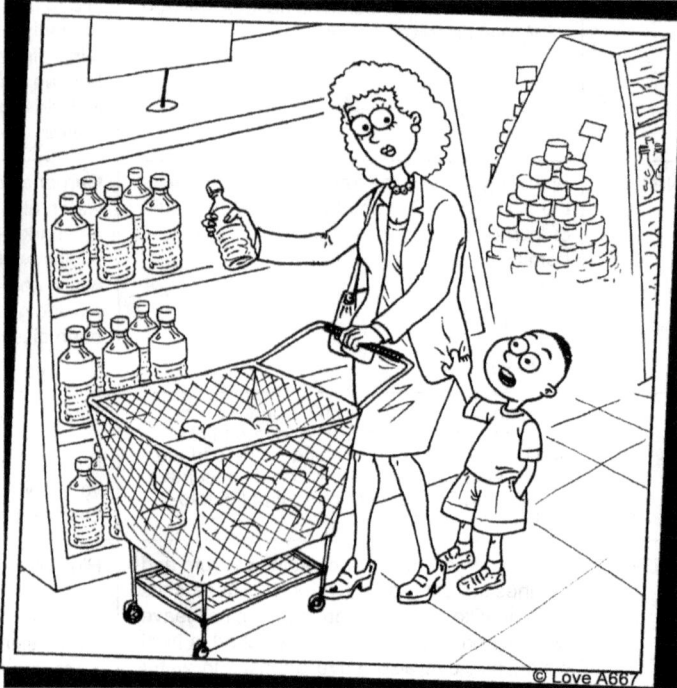

Snapshots at jasonlove.com

"How come we call it spring water
when they sell it all year long?"

drinking water with elevated risk and incidence of cancer. Many people now choose bottled water to avoid chemicals such as chlorine, contaminants, and bacteria. Many also choose bottled because it tastes better, and some can even distinguish tastes between different bottled waters. Yes, water apparently tastes different to different people, and some are more sensitive to chemical and chlorine tastes than others. In fact, popular water filter companies specifically market on this premise, making the claim: "Removes Chlorine Taste." But something in that claim still smells chlorinated. They make it sound as though they remove the chlorine, but beware: they only claimed to mask the chlorine taste.

There are, however, new filters with improved technology at more affordable prices. Whole house systems are typically very effective and filter all of the water in your house. Both counter-top and under-sink filters help assure clean water from a specific tap, most often placed in the kitchen and used for drinking, cooking, and washing dishes. Hand-held filters (about the size of a fountain pen) are available, too, for dining out.

Shower filters are also important. Unless you have a whole-house system, the water you are bathing and showering could be stressing your immune system and negatively impacting your health.

Jack and Jill's Guide to Keeping Your Head Above Water

✧ Avoid chlorinated water. This applies both to drinking and bathing.

✧ Check the source and purification methods used by your favorite bottled water.

✧ Be sure to drink enough high-quality, pure water.

✧ Don't be so afraid of "bad" water that you don't drink enough. Water is essential to our bodies!

We have all taken a long, hot shower, fogging up the mirror and filling the bathroom with steam. We breathe this steam into our lungs, and with the gaseous water molecules, chemicals like chlorine are going along for the ride. Chlorine also damages your hair and skin. A shower filter is an easy way to be proactive about your family's health while requiring minimal, if any, effort on a daily basis.

SILVER WATER

As previously mentioned, water has the ability to carry substances, both good and bad. One positive example is when a metal, such as silver, is prepared in a water solution. Silver has many beneficial properties, including being anti-bacterial, anti-fungal, anti-viral, as well as lending healing support to tissues of the body. It has been used for centuries as a medicine, and is commonly found today in health food stores. "Colloidal silver" is a product that comes from suspending silver particles (colloidal suspension) in purified water.

Although there are many safe, non-toxic uses of silver for health, manufacturing processes, quality, and proper dosage are especially important when using it. There have been unfortunate incidents in which the over-consumption of poorly manufactured silver colloids resulted in Argyria, a benign cosmetic condition, evidenced by a bluish tint to the skin. I don't care how much you loved the cartoon on TV, no one wants to be a "Smurf" in real life.

Fortunately, manufacturing standards and technology have improved dramatically, even leading to a new category of silver products, referred to as "silver hydrosols." In these products, both the quality and quantity of silver particles in ultra-pure water have been studied and formulated for both highest safety and effectiveness. Several conditions are currently being researched to show where silver hydrosol may be effective. One way to find out more is to cull information from the Immunogenic Research Foundation **www.imref.org.**

SILVER CONCENTRATION	RfD 1 teaspoon taken once a day	RfD Power dose: 1 teaspoon taken 5-7 times daily
10 ppm	50 mcg	250-350 mcg
25 ppm	125 mcg	625-878 mcg
50 ppm	250 mcg	1,250-1750 mcg
100 ppm	500 mcg	2,500-3,500 mcg
250 ppm	1,250 mcg	6,250-8,750 mcg
500 ppm	2,500 mcg	12,500-17,500 mcg
1,000 ppm	5,000 mcg	25,000-35,000 mcg
2,000 ppm	10,000 mcg	50,000-70,000 mcg

෴

WATER QUANTITY

How much water is too much, and how much is not enough? This depends, as each person is unique, and each day may have variables needing consideration. When it comes to quantity, your environment, lifestyle, activity level, and physiology are among the factors that determine your individual needs for H20. A person working outdoors on a hot, sunny, dry, day would perspire more and therefore require more hydration than someone in an air conditioned office building, working at a desk.

Most recommend 6-8 eight ounce glasses of water per day. See what works for you, given your size, environment, and level of exertion.

෴

LIQUID THOUGHTS

"What the Bleep Do We Know," a popular documentary about quantum physics, presents an experiment on water in which emotions and thoughts had an apparent effect on the molecular structure of water. More and more research is currently underway studying the structure of water, and any abilities to carry messages and substances, both harmful and beneficial.

WATER CURES

Water is not just a staple but also a cure. Water helps you detoxify your blood of toxins. Whether you're concerned about acne or wrinkles, water is essential–literally–to healthy skin!

Snapshots at jasonlove.com

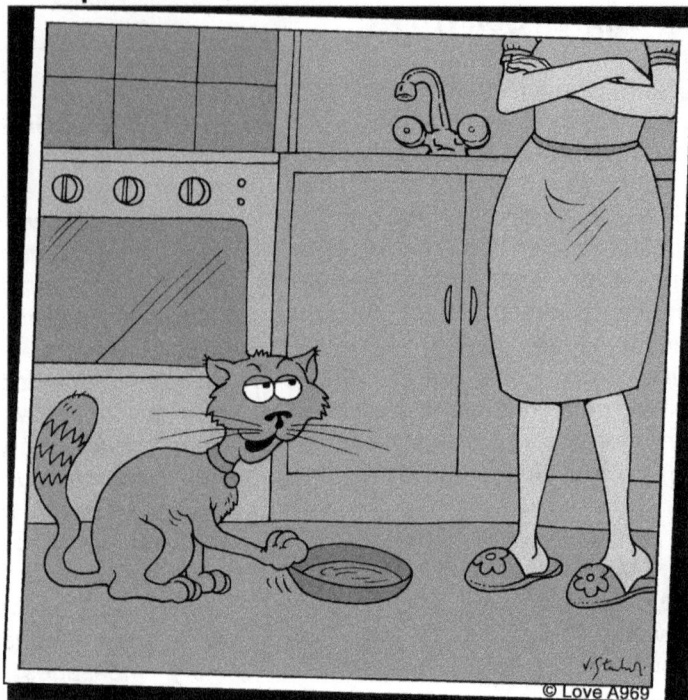

"Tap water?! As *if*."

Notes

CHAPTER 12

The Princess and the Pea
On a Good Night's Sleep

"It seldom happens that a man changes his life through his habitual reasoning. No matter how fully he may sense the new plans and aims revealed to him by reason, he continues to plod along in old paths until his life becomes frustrating and unbearable - he finally makes the change only when his usual life can no longer be tolerated."

- Leo Tolstoy

The poor princess was up all night because she had a small pea in her bed, under a stack of twenty mattresses and twenty featherbeds. While she only suffered one night of poor sleep and this "test" proved her to be nobility so the young prince would propose to her, long nights and sleep difficulties are more problematic for the rest of us.

Millions of people have trouble falling or staying asleep on a regular basis. The sales of sleep medications in the US are increasing at lightening speed. Then we don't understand why we are not feeling well. It may seem easy to take a pill just to knock yourself out at night, but more people are wondering why they are having such difficulty doing something so simple as sleeping.

❧

Nutrition

Caffeine, cake, cookies, and other sweets will interfere, at night with your sleep. If you drink caffeine, do it early in the day. If you need a late-night snack, choose something other than chocolate. But good nutrition for sleep is about more than what you eat right before bed. In fact, all of the health and dietary guidelines throughout this book contribute to a healthy, balanced body, which is certainly good for sleep. Eating well may not solve your sleep problem and if it does the results may not be immediate, but you will have a much harder time relaxing and getting the rest you need if your diet is keeping you off balance.

❦

STRESS

As mentioned in earlier chapters, stress causes the adrenal glands to produce a hormone called cortisol. Cortisol is known as the stress hormone, causing a "fight or flight" reaction in the body (heightened memory functions, quick, shallow breathing, muscles pumped and ready for action). This quick burst of energy is useful if you're running from a predator, but not when you're trying to sleep! When the stress response is over-activated, it's hard to return to normal functioning, let alone relax and drift away.

> ## $\subset$ TRESS AND AGING
>
> In Chinese medicine, the kidneys and adrenal glands are connected to the hair. It seems to make sense then, that as we stress out our body and deplete our mineral stores, our hair would be affected. This is why grey hair occurs in those dealing with a lot of stress.

In addition to sleep interference, higher and more prolonged levels of cortisol in the bloodstream (like those associated with chronic stress) have been shown to have negative effects, such as:

- Impaired cognitive performance
- Suppressed thyroid function
- Blood sugar imbalances, such as hyperglycemia
- Decreased bone density
- Decreased muscle tissue
- Higher blood pressure
- Lowered immunity and inflammatory responses in the body
- Increased abdominal fat

Excess abdominal fat has been associated with a greater number of health problems than fat deposited in other areas of the body. Health problems associated with increased stomach fat include heart attacks, stroke, higher levels of "bad" cholesterol (LDL) and lower levels of "good" cholesterol (HDL), which can lead to other health problems!

To keep cortisol levels healthy and under control, the body's relaxation response should be activated after the fight or flight response occurs. You can learn to relax your body with various stress management techniques, and you can make lifestyle changes in order to keep your body from reacting to stress in the first place. What changes can you make in your life and in your actions and reactions to reduce your overall stress levels?

Dietary De-Stressors

Adrenal glands are your key to managing stress hormones and your ability to handle stress in general. Along with eating foods full of minerals, such as dark green leafy vegetables and sea vegetables (dulse, nori, arame, hijiki, etc.), getting rid of refined table salt and replacing it with high-quality sea salt is also important, and simple to do. Herbs such as astragalus, ashwaganda, maca, and ginseng are called "adaptogens." This is because they help strengthen adrenal glands by adapting to the stress levels of your body. If you have been under a lot of stress, your adrenals may be working extra hard. These herbs will help support their function and make sure they don't burn out. On the other hand, perhaps you have already burned out those tiny, yet important glands sitting on top of the kidneys. These same herbs adapt and help to rebuild the adrenals, so you can continue to handle normal stress. Look for formulas that combine a few of these different herbs together, as many herbalists feel that the synergy of the herbs work better together than individually.

> Stress levels continue to escalate in every age group.
>
> Stress has been linked to all leading causes of death: heart disease, cancer, lung ailments, accidents, cirrhosis, and suicide.
>
> 75-90% of all visits to primary care physicians are for stress-related complaints or disorders.

A good B-vitamin complex is great for energy and supporting many of the body's regular functions. Some people have a hard time digesting B vitamin supplements. If you do, you may want to look for a form that has been somewhat predigested, or in an "active", co-enzyme form, suggesting easier absorption and greater potency.

Mind Shifts for Stress Relief

If you're under a great deal of stress, you may have more of a stress problem than a sleep issue. It could be one large stress or perhaps many little stressors that are disrupting your sleep patterns. Stress is inevitable, but also somewhat manageable. It could come in the form of something small, like a pea under the mattress making you uncomfortable, like in the Princess and the Pea fairytale, or something devastating, even life altering. You may need help getting through a tough time; many of us do. A pill may help you get some sleep tonight so you can be somewhat alert in the morning meeting, but if you don't take steps to get to the root of stress in your life, even sadness, your sleep problem will probably persist. Sleep deprivation itself becomes a stress, perpetuating a downward spiral. So don't stress over getting enough sleep; that stress can interfere with your efforts to sleep! As ironic as this may sound, it does happen.

---

*T*he Princess's Guide to the Royal Treatment You Deserve

✧ Get plenty of rest. Your body heals and repairs while you sleep.

✧ Try not to go to bed with any food in your stomach. (Wait at least two hours after eating. The body won't be able to rest if it has to work to digest food while you sleep.)

✧ Practice yoga, tai chi, meditation, deep breathing exercises, or visit an acupuncturist. (Most of these practices are rooted in thousands of years of experience and have documented health benefits.)

✧ Eat, sleep, and be merry—and don't stress out over a little thing like a pea!

Learn to let go of the little things. Celebrate life. From major events to little, quickly fleeting moments. It is not easy, and stress never disappears completely. Taoism suggests that circumstances fall into two categories: those we can control and those we cannot control. The more you recognize and let go of the things you cannot control, the more time and energy you will have to focus on the things you can control. You start to better manage and cope with stresses by accepting that some things are bigger than us and out of our control. This is considered a step along the path to enlightenment in Taoism, as well as an important step towards a healthier ever after.

∽

MORE TIPS FOR BETTER SLEEP

Natural products that may help with sleep often contain melatonin, valerian root, passionflower, or magnesium. Recently popular, an amino acid called L-theanine has been shown beneficial not only for sleep, but for stress in general.

Some quick, basic tips for better sleep include:

- Turn off the TV, or at least set a sleep timer.
- Read or listen to mellow music before bed.
- Practice deep breathing exercises.
- Avoid food for at least 1-2 hrs before going to lie down.
- Avoid substances that interfere with sleep cycles: sugar, caffeine, and artificial chemicals.
- Try some aromatherapy.

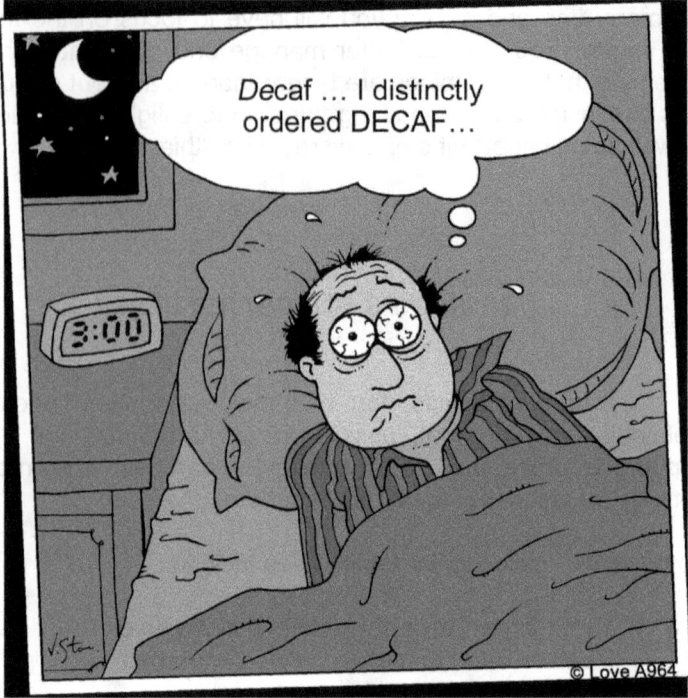

Notes

CHAPTER 13

⤖

The Old Woman Who Lived in a Shoe

A Tight Fit

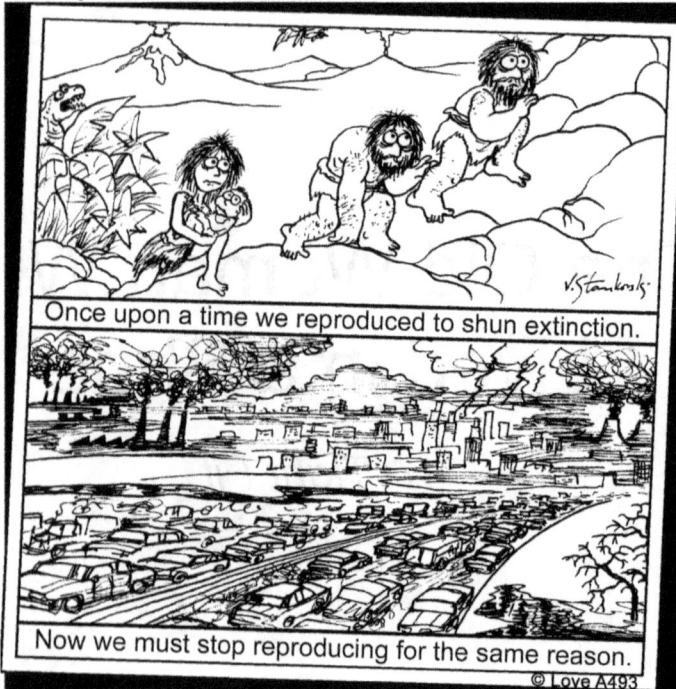

"There was an old woman who lived in a shoe. She had so many children, she didn't know what to do."

With overpopulation [3] continuing to crowd us in, the old woman is not the only one suffering a lack of space and the destruction caused by overcrowding. We are currently in the midst of a slow, but purposeful shift in the way we look at our health, our lifestyles, and the world around us, our ecosystem.

☙

GOING GREEN

Being "green" is not some out-there hippie-only concept. It's about being health conscious, maintaining optimism, and making an effort to care a little bit about simple things, like community, family, the environment, and evolving as a society. This is being holistic. New and recycled materials are being used in industrial design, from recycled rubber sidewalks to solar panels, and the future holds great potential.

---

[3] US population: According to the US census, the approximate US Population is currently a little over 300 million, nearly double the number of people back in 1950. In 1900, the US population was only 76 million.

Veggie Craze

Why are so many people becoming vegetarian? And why is it wise to at least cut down our meat consumption? Some great books and websites that offer perspective and background on factory farming and the impact of meat-heavy diets on people, animals, and the environment can be found below:

⟡ Ishmael: "An Adventure of the Mind and Spirit", Daniel Quinn, Bantam/Turner Books, 1992.

⟡ The Food Revolution: "How Your Diet Can Help Save Your Life and Our World", John Robbins, Conari Press, 2001.

⟡ The China Study: "The Most Comprehensive Study of Nutrition Ever Conducted and the Startling Implications for Diet, Weight Loss and Long-term Health", by T. Colin Campbell, Thomas M. Campbell II, John Robbins, Benbella Books, 2006.

⟡ Appetite for Profit: "How the Food Industry Undermines Our Health and How to Fight Back", Michele Simon, Nation Books, 2006.

⟡ http://www.EarthSave.org

⟡ http://www.PCRM.org
(the website of the Physicians Committee for Responsible Medicine)

That is, of course, if we collectively make an effort and make better choices, ones that respect and care for the planet.

Forms of energy like solar, hydro (water), and wind power are being integrated into more functional tools. Hybrid cars, natural gas options, and even biodiesel (a renewable diesel fuel made from natural products, such as soybean oil) are becoming more available. Not only does biodiesel help with our fuel needs, it also supports local farmers and brings us back to agriculture, the roots of our civilization.

❧

EAT YOUR VEGGIES!

We already talked about the internal effects of eating large amounts of meat; excessive meat consumption is hard on the external environment, as well. The way animals are raised has been modified to keep up with the demand. Rain forests and other important natural environments are cleared to provide more land for raising cattle. This now has an impact on the planet and can even be related to the global warming issues. Animals are horribly mistreated in factory farms and pumped with antibiotics and hormones to make more animal protein available for the supermarkets.

"The China Study," a book by Dr. T. Colin Campbell, is based on a 20-year study of various diseases and lifestyle factors in Taiwan and rural China. Now commonly known as "The China Study," as the book title suggests, the project was a collaborative research effort among Dr. Campbell, Cornell University, Oxford University, and the Chinese Academy of Preventative Medicine. This investigation into both nutritional and social influences opened a much-needed discussion about health and wellness. Their research found that those consuming a plant-based diet were healthier than those who incorporated animal proteins.

Although there is evidence that a vegetarian diet may be beneficial for both the health of individuals and the planet, I don't believe that we all will (or should) become vegetarians. However, in comparison to the standard American diet, we should definitely be incorporating more fresh fruits and vegetables. Incorporating more plant-based nutrition and whole foods into your diet is vital for maintaining optimal health.

Arsenic is a common additive in factory chicken feed. It has been used for the past fifty years and continues to be used to kill parasites and promote growth.

Less than 1% of the Earth's water is usable for human consumption.

About 25 million pounds of antibiotics are fed to US livestock every year.

America's farmed animals produce 1.3 billion tons of waste per year. One cow alone produces 100 pounds per day. Manure is one of our most common water pollutants.

The world feeds nearly 43% of all harvested grain to animals to produce meat. Imagine if those grains, or at least a percentage, were used to feed the approximately 800 million people who live with chronic hunger or save the approximately 16,000 children who die from hunger-related causes.

Source: 101 Reasons Why I'm a Vegetarian (7th edition), Pamela Rice, 2007.

(Available as a full-length book from Lantern Books or PDF from http://www.vivavegie.org/101)

Again, I'm not a vegetarian. I am a "conscious consumer"; a citizen of the globe as we all are. When we make choices, we have to look at the big picture and realize that even small choices have a large impact.

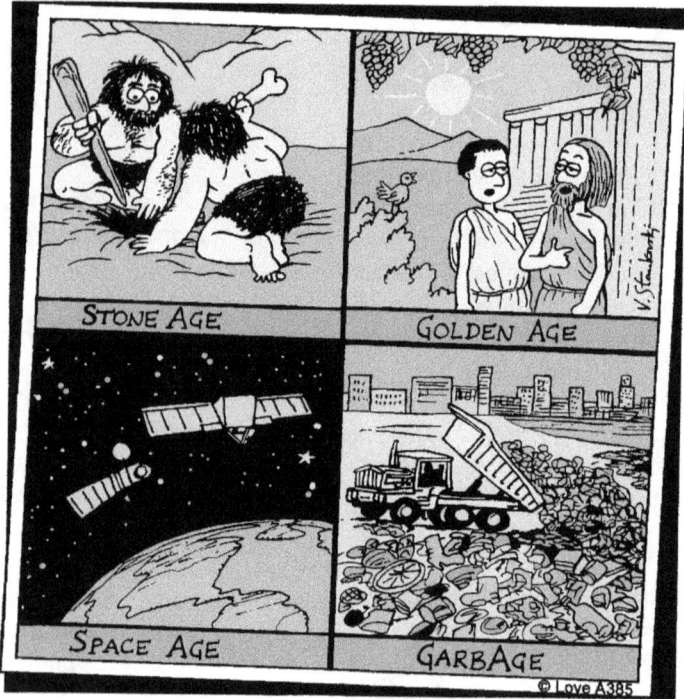

Snapshots at jasonlove.com

Notes

CHAPTER 14

꧁⸱⫻⸱꧂

The Jetsons

Into the Future

*"**O**ur home food dispenser broke, and I had to wait 20 seconds at the check out counter. Such inefficiency!"* - Jane Jetson

The television show (which originated in the '60s and was brought back with popular success in the '80s) was set in the late 21st century and featured encyclopedias stored on objects the size of cigarette lighters and people speaking to each other on "visaphones," telephones with video. People also lived in skypads, far above the natural order of things and ate most of their food in pill form. They had transcended nature altogether, a vision of the future that many would like to believe because it's easy and clean and negates our need to be responsible for the planet. But no matter how much technological innovations take us away from nature and even assist us in maintaining health, we will never completely outsmart nature!

❧

MODERN-DAY NUTRITION

Traditional cultures that lived in balance with nature, eating natural foods, have historically been healthier and lived much longer than we do in the US today. In fact, the "standard American diet" is also known as SAD, and we can see the physical and emotional toll it has had on us. This move to quicker, modified, nuked, trans-fatty foods has not been progressive; it has been regressive. But we do live in today's world, and even the purest eaters among us are taking in fewer nutrients because the soil is so depleted. Food contains both macronutrients (proteins, carbohydrates, fats, etc.) and micronutrients (vitamins, minerals, antioxidants, etc.) The levels of these nutrients have dramatically decreased in the food we grow today, a result of poor care of the soil, environmental toxins, sped up growing cycles, and truck-ripened produce.

Fruits and vegetables, whole grains, nuts and seeds, have been a source of nutrition since the beginning of mankind. Unfortunately, our overzealous attempt to emulate nature using science and technology has led to a gross abuse of the land and its many gifts. We now face the obvious challenge of re-assessing our situation and working to find a balance between science and nature.

There is hope. Actually, there is good news. Innovative new products and a more open minded scientific community are helping to provide the best possible solutions to address our health needs.

⁐

NUTRITIONAL DENSITY

Is there a difference

TRACE MINERALS

Many trace minerals are important for health and impact us every day—even if we have never heard of them. Boron, for example, has been depleted from the soil, our food, and our bodies, but research shows that Boron:

Helps strengthen and optimize bone and joint health.

Regulates metabolism of minerals, such as calcium, and subsequently bone and cartilage metabolism.

Impacts steroid hormone levels.

Improves the body's ability to heal wounds.

If Boron affects all of those things (and more), imagine how a deficiency of this or other trace minerals can impact your health on a day-to-day basis.

Sources: Naghi (1993), Nielsen, (1992), Benderdour (2000)

between the nutritional content of conventional versus organic produce? Is it worth the money? YES!

We are all walking around today malnourished. Even the more health conscious of consumers often rely only on food for nourishment. Research shows that there is a nutritional difference between conventional and organic fruits and vegetables. Organic fruit may not look as bright and big as some of its conventional counterparts (engineered to grow bigger, faster, and more colorful), but looks aren't everything. In fact, when it comes to nutrition and even taste, it may be like buying a well-packaged, brightly colored, box of hot air. The food is not very satisfying to your taste buds, or to your body's nutritional requirements.

The body is a machine that needs fuel to run. You know you don't get the same performance from 86-grade fuel as you would 94. You could say that it is more concentrated power. So you eat, and sure it fills your stomach, but it doesn't satisfy your body. So, the body is stressed and wants more nutrients. It tells you to keep eating. You eat more. Lots of empty calories are converted and stored because the body

Sweet Discoveries: *GLYCONUTRIENTS*

Protein is made up of chains of amino acids. The amino acids are the "building blocks" of proteins. Fats are made up from fatty acids coming together. Some are essential, meaning they are important, but the body does not make them and needs to get them from your diet. Recently, eight simple sugars were identified to be components that act as the building blocks of carbohydrates. These mono (one) saccharides (sugars)— also known as glyconutrients—help to maintain health and enhance cell-to-cell communication in the body. Research suggests that these sugars are extremely important for immune function, but seem to be quite deficient in our modern diet. These eight glyconutrients are: Mannose, Fucose, Xylose, Galactose, Glucose, N-acetylglucosamine, N-acetylneuraminic acid (sialic acid), and N-acetylgalactosamine. Glyconutrients are recognized as being relatively absent in our modern American diets, just as we lack many vitamins, minerals, and other vital nutrients. Emerging science strongly suggests that supplementation of these glyconutrients can support healthy glucose metabolism, enhance the immune system, and help promote a greater health and sense of well being overall. Derived from natural sources such as aloe plants and certain fruits and vegetables, glyconutrients are important to the story of a healthier ever after.

starts to worry about whether it will ever get real nourishment again.

Another analogy is gold. Pure gold is 24k. An ounce of 24k gold is worth a lot more than an ounce of 14k gold. Same weight, but the purity, the density of the gold is more in the 24k. If we compare this to food, I believe that most conventional, processed food is like fool's gold–it

Support Companies that are cGMP!

Check to see that the vitamin manufacturers are cGMP (certified for Good Manufacturing Practices) and that they are operating in a conscious way. This means that they are using green energy and even making changes to their packaging materials to be more environmentally friendly. These factors may seem small or insignificant, but even one small step in the right direction is progress, and our individual choices have a global impact!

SNAPSHOTS at jasonlove.com

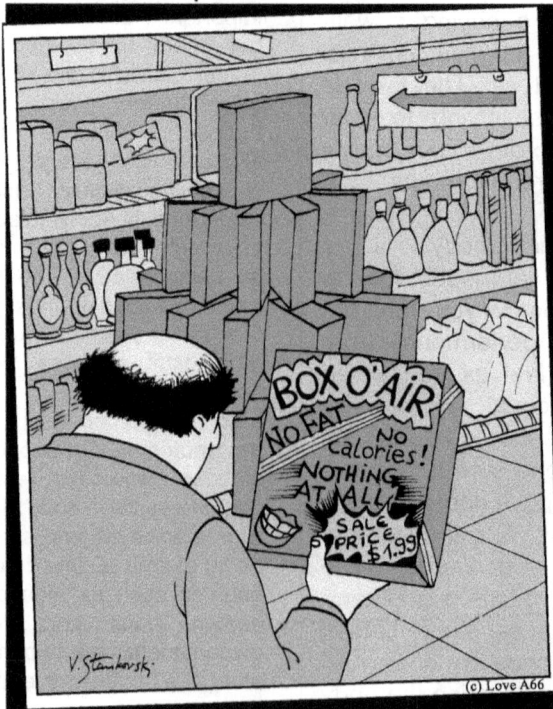

looks similar, but fool's gold has almost no value, as compared to the real stuff. Some conventional food does have value, but the quality is 14k at best, and not even solid. It's gold-plated, looking good on the surface, but nutritionally hollow. Organic food is more like solid 18k-24k gold. Your body wants the good stuff! The better the purity and density, the more efficiently the body will be fueled and health optimized. Ideally natural fruits and vegetables should make up about 70-80% of your daily diet. Unfortunately, the average diet today seems to have 20-30% at best.

∽

NUTRITION PYRAMID

FOOD, the foundation of the pyramid and most regular source of nourishment, has been discussed throughout this book. You eat every day, several times a day, just about every day of your life. You may have heard of the saying, "You are what you eat." Think about it. Such a large percentage of your life involves and revolves around food. For some, this concept needs to be taken more seriously, as the choices we make about food affect all aspects of our life. Eating fresh, nutrient dense food, which is preferably organic, will help build a strong foundation to your personal nutrition pyramid.

After food, the category of **SUPPLEMENTS** enters the spotlight. "But I don't like taking pills," you say, or maybe you just don't remember to take them.

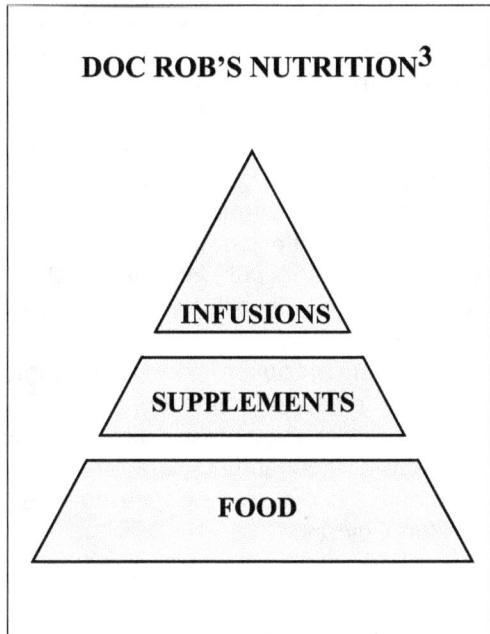

DOC ROB'S NUTRITION[3]

INFUSIONS

SUPPLEMENTS

FOOD

Do you own a great collection of half empty pill bottles, cluttering up your cabinet? A key point to remember is, the less nutrition you get from what you eat, the more important it becomes to get nutrients from pills, liquids, powders, etc. The good news is, today more than ever you have many options, from form to flavor, so that investing in some quality natural products, preferably whole-food based, has become not only easier, but tastier too. Some people like to make a drink from fresh squeezed fruits and vegetables, or maybe a shake in the morning, throwing everything in to it but the kitchen sink. Some carry protein bars, and others, a small pillbox, remembering to take their vitamins and minerals with their meals. (Don't forget those digestive enzymes!) Incorporating quality supplements into your day will help add valuable nutrients to your pyramid, helping build on whatever food foundation you choose to have. Remember, in the end, it is always your choice.

What if you can't or won't eat healthier, and don't want to be bothered constantly with taking pills and powders? Does that mean there is no hope? Of course not, life is full of options. You just need to take the time to learn what they are. Regardless of what you hear on the news, or what the latest diet tries to convince you of, it is ridiculous to think you can eat perfectly. There is no such thing as the perfect diet, perfect weight, perfect pill, or even perfect health. Maybe you are choosing to eat well, and taking supplements, but still don't feel like you are getting all the nutrition your body needs. Many people today have such stressed out lives and imbalanced digestive systems, that the body doesn't absorb the nutrients from the food they eat, or supplements they ingest. This is where the third component to the nutrition pyramid comes in. Nutrient **INFUSIONS**, or I.V.'s, play a major role and offer an effective way to bypass the digestive system, delivering nutrients right into the blood. Of course, some people don't want anything to do with needles, it's not for every day, and you need a licensed, trained health professional to administer the infusion, but it is definitely an option worth looking into. Nutrient infusions can be utilized to increase your energy, help you recover more quickly from illness, and may even make it easier to lose some weight, providing that little extra nutritional fuel you aren't getting from food or supplements. For many, it is the icing on their nutrient dense cake, the cap to their nutritional pyramid.

We all have different lives, lifestyles, and preferences. It is not one or the other, all or nothing. Work to figure out what combination of Food, Supplements, and Infusions works best for you, for your lifestyle. That is what is unique and great about the Nutrition[3] Pyramid: there is no set program or diet to follow. Continue to learn and make better choices about your health, and a healthier ever after can be yours.

⟨∽⟩

SUPPLEMENTS

Though we haven't entered a future where pills replace food, we have entered one where supplements are necessary to ensure total nutrition. Scientists have isolated and replicated specific nutrients to address individual deficiencies or health concerns. Although this is quite useful, most people who realize the importance of taking some form of supplement prefer to take a product that offers multi-nutrient vitamins, minerals, anti-oxidants, amino-acids, glyconutrients, etc—all at once. While isolated nutrients may be very good for specific conditions, when looking for a daily multi-nutrient, the best form of daily supplement is whole-food based.

Whole Food Based Supplements

Many scientific advances are amazing! We are learning more about nutrients than ever before, and the quality of vitamins is changing, offering supplements that are closer than ever before to whole foods and more evidence of their effectiveness. Whole food based supplements are made from concentrated, whole fruits, vegetables, and superfoods. Tests are showing the positive effects these functional-food-based vitamins have on physiology, and the way the body functions. There is now scientific proof that

---

Fermentation & Vitamins

A new trend is applying the fermentation process in making supplements to liberate the nutrients for optimal absorption. Supplements that use this process are not common at this point, but worth seeking out. The benefits of fermentation still apply when food is transformed into supplements!

taking these multi-vitamins is benefiting your health! Because this approach to formulation is cutting edge, not all products and companies have caught up, but be sure that your multi is keeping up with these exciting nutritional advances.

So what do you do about it? Do you still go out like so many people and buy any cheap bottle that says "MULTI" or "ONE A DAY" on it, blindly hoping that the daily doses will provide you with some nourishment? Or do you make a conscious choice and try to find something that has been researched and shown to contribute to health? Good, proven supplements are a valuable investment in your health. They still support your healthy diet and help pick up the nutritional slack when you go non-organic or processed or even choose fast food from time to time. There are now convenient ways to get custom, personalized vitamin formulas made specifically for you and your nutrient needs!

Three-a-Day

Although ideal, it is very difficult to get all the basic nutrients our body needs, compressed into one pill. Some popular manufacturers claim to offer everything in a one-a-day pill, but they have to overly compress nutrients in the effort. For many people, especially those with digestive issues, the pill never breaks apart and no nutrients are absorbed. Some one-a-day supplements are surely better than others, but it's better to take whole food supplements, and take them with each meal.

The Four Vitamin Essentials

When choosing a vitamin, look for the following:

1. Food ingredients are organic (most, if not all).

2. Fruits and vegetables are harvested and stored in a way that nutrient potency is maintained (usually flash frozen).

3. Vitamins are not condensed into one-a-day formulas. (They are best when not super-condensed, and should be taken and absorbed spread out through the day, with meals.)

4. It is not just the quantity (% daily value) of vitamins that

is important, but also the quality. The human body often recognizes/absorbs food-based ingredients more effectively than the isolated, man-made ingredients. Isolated nutrients can be useful for treating specific deficiencies or health conditions, but basic nutrition should start with food and food-based supplements.

Nutrient Infusions

Notice that the food pyramid is capped by "Nutrient Infusions." As discussed, a large percentage of our society requires some additional nutritional support. I.V. (intravenous therapy) nutrient infusions deliver fluids, nutrients, and medications directly into the blood stream, bypassing the digestive tract and providing an almost immediate source of nutrients for the body to use. Nutrient infusions have been shown to alleviate symptoms in numerous health conditions, including fibromyalgia and chronic fatigue. Nutrient infusions are even great when fatigued, feeling under the weather, or recovering from a late night out. I also believe that nutrient infusions can be a major asset in the fight against obesity.

Not to be depended on exclusively, but along with eating high quality, nutrient dense food (preferably in small portions throughout the day) and supplementing your diet with a whole food multi-nutrient that is made from real food (at least once a day), it may also prove to be useful to incorporate a multi-nutrient infusion into your lifestyle. For treatment of specific conditions, once a week or more may be recommended, whereas one or two infusions per month might provide nutrients for a more pro-active, preventative approach. Nutrient infusions are fairly popular among naturopathic doctors, but any licensed medical professional should be able to offer this service. More and more people are beginning to understand the concept of nutritional density, and as they make a conscious effort to optimize their intake of quality nutrients, the likelihood of dis-ease should dramatically go down.

⌒୨

VISIONS OF A HEALTHY FUTURE

The ideal future is not space cars and Venus vacations that take us further from the earth that fortifies us. The future is here and now in creating a nutrient plan that combines mining the 24k gold resources left in our soil with whole food supplements–protecting our natural resources– keeping ourselves grounded–and returning our attention to this precious Earth.

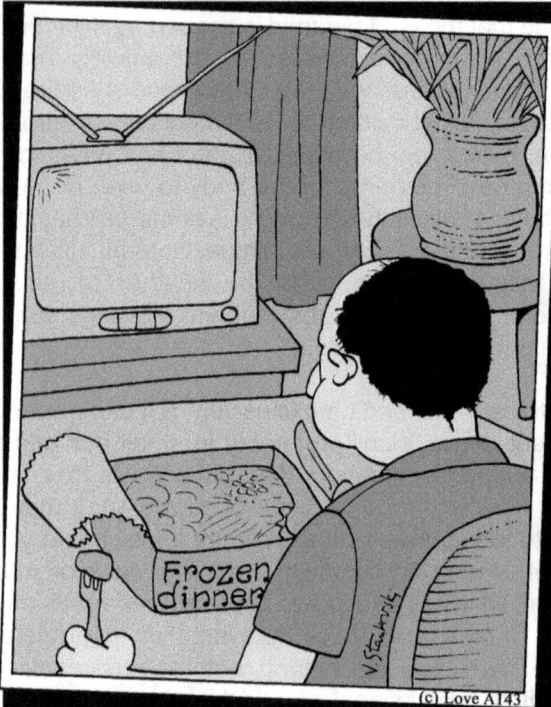

Three square meals a day.

Notes

CHAPTER IS

~·//~

Happily Ever After

"You don't get to choose how you're going to die, or when. You can only decide how you're going to live now."
- Joan Baez

T his is your story, even though you didn't get to choose the opening setting or write all of the scenes. You are not only the main character of this tale that is your life, but you get to create much of the story and make choices that will lead you to a happier, healthier ever after.

Finding your way to A Healthier Ever After begins with making small changes, trying them out and seeing how you feel. While it is impossible to control everything, getting into the habit of making better choices, concentrating on the few things you actually can control, will improve the quality of your life. If "quality of life" to you means never making any sacrifices and making every choice based on immediate desires, you're missing the bigger storyline.

When you integrate healthier food choices, exercise, and relaxation, working towards more balance in your life, you can actually enjoy your life more fully, as you will have more energy, be happier, and feel a greater sense of well-being.

Healthier Ever After Reminders

- Eat healthful meals and snacks.
- Incorporate high-quality supplements.

155

- Eat more fresh foods than processed.
- Choose organic products when possible.
- Eat smaller meals more often.
- Minimize your exposure to a toxic environment. (That means clean water for drinking, cooking, and showering; clean air; non-toxic cleaning supplies in the home; and chemical-free personal care products and makeup.)
- Avoid cigarettes (always) and try to cut back on alcohol.
- Make an appointment with a naturopathic doctor (http://www. naturopathic.org) to help you assess your health and set a course for a long, happy and healthy ever after.
- Celebrate life!

This is your unique story, and no two characters in this world are exactly the same. Your friends might try a new supplement of food that makes them feel great, and the same thing might have little or no effect on you. Or maybe something works wonderfully for you for a while, and then your body needs a change. Listen to your body, find a health care practitioner who listens to you, be a conscious consumer, and be open to new ideas while staying in tune with what feels right for you in the end.

Happily, we can choose to live A Healthier Ever After.
And you will live Happily, Healthfully, Ever After.

❧

The End

The best compliment to a child or a friend is the feeling you give him that he has been set free to make his own inquiries, to come to conclusions that are right for him, whether or not they coincide with your own." - Alistair Cooke

Conscious Consumers Listen!

Critical listening is an essential skill for the conscious consumer. A new listening book by Linda Eve Diamond, RULE #1: STOP TALKING! A Guide to Listening, addresses "listening in the age of overload" and offers insights into how to become a "savvy listener." With all of the conflicting information coming at us, this book is a great guide to breaking through the confusion, listening to discern what is true, and asking good questions.

Notes

Health
Designed
with YOU
in mind

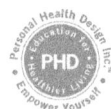

PHD™

Personal Health Design, Inc.

Visit www.PHDunlimited.com.

Sign up for your free 1 year

Preferred Membership!

PHD

Personal Health Design Inc.™

Education for Healthier Living

Empower Yourself

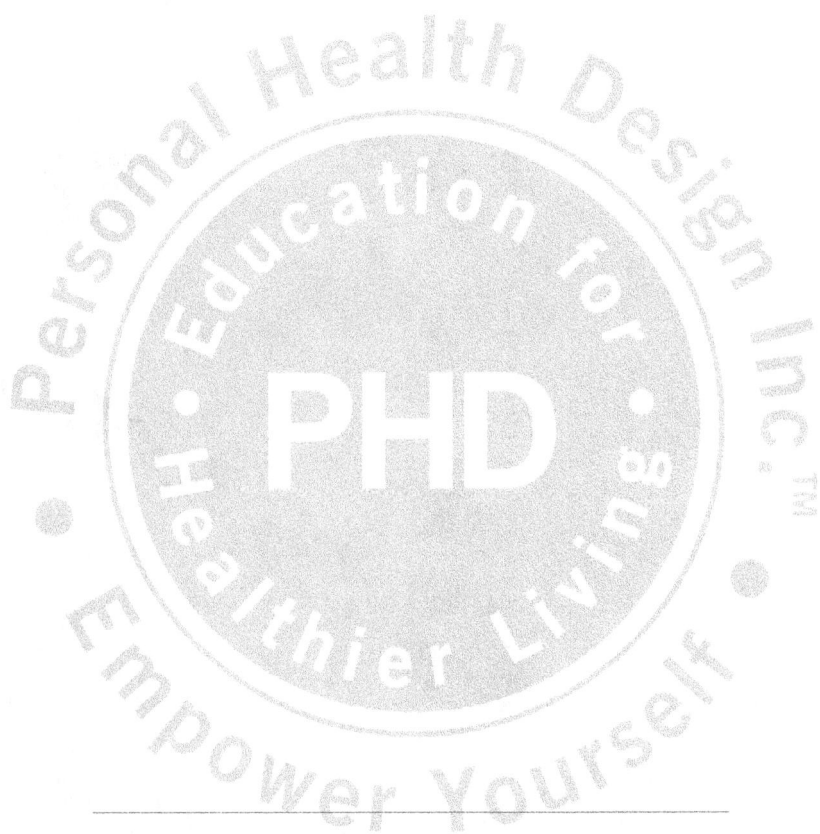

www.PHDunlimited.com	**fyi@PHDunlimited.com**

Corporate	602.321.8251	Toll Free	866.650.3200
Fax	602.532.7505		

NEW YORK	Manhattan Brooklyn	**ILLINOIS** **ARIZONA**	Chicago Scottsdale
FLORIDA	Boca Raton Hollywood Miami	**CALIFORNIA**	Santa Monica Beverly Hills San Diego

References

Aggarwal, R., J. Sentz, and M. A. Miller. "Role of zinc administration in prevention of childhood diarrhea and respiratory illnesses: a meta-analysis." Pediatrics 119.6 (2007): 1120-30.

Albano, H., et al. "Characterization of two bacteriocins produced by Pediococcus acidilactici isolated from "Alheira", a fermented sausage traditionally produced in Portugal." Int.J.Food Microbiol. 116.2 (2007): 239-47.

Ammerman, A., et al. "Efficacy of interventions to modify dietary behavior related to cancer risk." Evid.Rep.Technol.Assess.(Summ.).25 (2000): 1-4.

Avena, N. M., P. Rada, and B. G. Hoebel. "Evidence for sugar addiction: Behavioral and neurochemical effects of intermittent, excessive sugar intake." Neurosci.Biobehav.Rev. (2007).

Balk, E., et al. "B vitamins and berries and age-related neurodegenerative disorders." Evid.Rep.Technol.Assess.(Full.Rep.).134 (2006): 1-161.

Becker, K. G. "Autism, asthma, inflammation, and the hygiene hypothesis." Med.Hypotheses (2007).

Bornet, F. R., et al. "Glycaemic response to foods: Impact on satiety and long-term weight regulation." Appetite (2007).

Boucher, B. J. "Inadequate vitamin D status: does it contribute to the disorders comprising syndrome 'X'?" Br.J.Nutr. 79.4 (1998): 315-27.

Bowen, J., M. Noakes, and P. M. Clifton. "Appetite hormones and energy intake in obese men after consumption of fructose, glucose and whey protein beverages." Int.J.Obes.(Lond) (2007).

Butel, M. J., et al. "Conditions of bifidobacterial colonization in preterm infants: a prospective analysis." J.Pediatr.Gastroenterol.Nutr. 44.5 (2007): 577-82.

Campbell, K. J., et al. "Associations between the home food environment and obesity-promoting eating behaviors in adolescence." Obesity. (Silver.Spring) 15.3 (2007): 719-30.

Cannell, J. J., et al. "Epidemic influenza and vitamin D." Epidemiol.Infect. 134.6 (2006): 1129-40.

---. "Epidemic influenza and vitamin D." Epidemiol.Infect. 134.6 (2006): 1129-40.

Chrysohoou, C., et al. "Long-term fish consumption is associated with protection against arrhythmia in healthy persons in a Mediterranean region--the ATTICA study." Am.J.Clin.Nutr. 85.5 (2007): 1385-91.

Collado, M. C., et al. "Potential probiotic characteristics of Lactobacillus and Enterococcus strains isolated from traditional dadih fermented milk against pathogen intestinal colonization." J.Food Prot. 70.3 (2007): 700-05.

Curtis, C. L., et al. "n-3 fatty acids specifically modulate catabolic factors involved in articular cartilage degradation." J.Biol.Chem. 275.2 (2000): 721-24.

Diamond, Linda Eve. Rule #1: Stop Talking!: A Guide to Listening. Listeners Press, 2007

Galloway, A. T., et al. "'Finish your soup': counterproductive effects of pressuring children to eat on intake and affect." Appetite 46.3 (2006): 318-23.

Garn, H. and H. Renz. "Epidemiological and immunological evidence for the hygiene hypothesis." Immunobiology 212.6 (2007): 441-52.

Gilhooly, C. H., et al. "Food cravings and energy regulation: the characteristics of craved foods and their relationship with eating behaviors and weight change during 6 months of dietary energy restriction." Int.J.Obes. (Lond) (2007).

Goldsobel, AB. "Risk of Celiac Disease Autoimmunity and Timing of Gluten Introduction in the Diet of Infants at Increased Risk of Disease." Pediatrics 118.Supplement (2006): S14-S15.

Haley, S, et al. "Sweetener Consumption in the United States: Distribution by Demographic and Product Characteristics." USDA Economic Research Service Outlook Report No. (SSS243-01) (2005).

Helland, I. B., et al. "Maternal supplementation with very-long-chain n-3 fatty acids during pregnancy and lactation augments children's IQ at 4 years of age." Pediatrics 111.1 (2003): e39-e44.

Hill, A. J. "The psychology of food craving." Proc.Nutr.Soc. 66.2 (2007): 277-85.

Hlebowicz, J., et al. "Effect of cinnamon on postprandial blood glucose, gastric emptying, and satiety in healthy subjects." Am.J.Clin.Nutr. 85.6 (2007): 1552-56.

Janson, C., et al. "The effect of infectious burden on the prevalence of atopy and respiratory allergies in Iceland, Estonia, and Sweden." J.Allergy Clin.Immunol. (2007).

Kidd, P. M. "Attention deficit/hyperactivity disorder (ADHD) in children: rationale for its integrative management." Altern.Med.Rev. 5.5 (2000): 402-28.

Knight, J. A., et al. "Vitamin D and reduced risk of breast cancer: a population-based case-control study." Cancer Epidemiol. Biomarkers Prev. 16.3 (2007): 422-29.

---. "Vitamin D and reduced risk of breast cancer: a population-based case-control study." Cancer Epidemiol.Biomarkers Prev. 16.3 (2007): 422-29.

Kobayashi, M., et al. "Promotive effect of Shoyu polysaccharides from soy sauce on iron absorption in animals and humans." Int.J.Mol.Med. 18.6 (2006): 1159-63.

Kouris-Blazos, A. and M. L. Wahlqvist. "Health economics of weight management: evidence and cost." Asia Pac.J.Clin.Nutr. 16 Suppl 1 (2007): 329-38.

Lakka, T. A. and D. E. Laaksonen. "Physical activity in prevention and treatment of the metabolic syndrome." Appl.Physiol Nutr.Metab 32.1 (2007): 76-88.

Linday, L. A., et al. "Effect of daily cod liver oil and a multivitamin-mineral supplement with selenium on upper respiratory tract pediatric visits by young, inner-city, Latino children: randomized pediatric sites." Ann.Otol.Rhinol.Laryngol. 113.11 (2004): 891-901.

Lumeng, Julie. "What Can We Do To Prevent Childhood Obesity?" Zero to Three (2005): 13-19.

Maclean, C. H., et al. "Effects of omega-3 fatty acids on cognitive function with aging, dementia, and neurological diseases." Evid.Rep. Technol. Assess.(Summ.).114 (2005): 1-3.

Mourao, D. M., et al. "Effects of food form on appetite and energy intake in lean and obese young adults." Int.J.Obes.(Lond) (2007).

Obihara, C. C., J. L. Kimpen, and N. Beyers. "The potential of Mycobacterium to protect against allergy and asthma." Curr.Allergy Asthma Rep.7.3 (2007): 223-30.

Olafsdottir, A. S., et al. "Relationship between dietary intake of cod liver oil in early pregnancy and birthweight." BJOG. 112.4 (2005): 424-29.

Pappa, H. M., et al. "Vitamin D status in children and young adults with inflammatory bowel disease." Pediatrics 118.5 (2006): 1950-61.

Perkin, M. R. "Unpasteurized milk: health or hazard?" Clin.Exp.Allergy 37.5 (2007): 627-30.

Qin, X. "High incidence of inflammatory bowel disease with improved hygiene and failure to get human-like IBD in laboratory animals." World J.Gastroenterol. 13.23 (2007): 3271.

Raeder, M. B., et al. "Associations between cod liver oil use and symptoms of depression: The Hordaland Health Study." J.Affect.Disord. 101.1-3 (2007): 245-49.

---. "Associations between cod liver oil use and symptoms of depression: The Hordaland Health Study." J.Affect.Disord. 101.1-3 (2007): 245-49.

Rampello, A., et al. "Effect of aerobic training on walking capacity and maximal exercise tolerance in patients with multiple sclerosis: a randomized crossover controlled study." Phys.Ther. 87.5 (2007): 545-55.

Ranji SR, et al. "Antibiotic Prescribing Behavior." Closing the Quality Gap: A Critical Analysis of Quality Improvement Strategies. 4 (2006).

Rizzello, C. G., et al. "Highly Efficient Gluten Degradation by Lactobacilli and Fungal Proteases during Food Processing: New Perspectives for Celiac Disease." Appl.Environ.Microbiol. 73.14 (2007): 4499-507.

Romagnani, S. "Coming back to a missing immune deviation as the main ex planatory mechanism for the hygiene hypothesis." J.Allergy Clin.Immunol. 119.6 (2007): 1511-13.

Ross, C. M. "Fish oil versus cod liver oil: is vitamin D a reason to go back to the future." J.Am.Board Fam.Pract. 18.5 (2005): 445-46.

Roxas, M. and J. Jurenka. "Colds and influenza: a review of diagnosis and conventional, botanical, and nutritional considerations." Altern.Med. Rev. 12.1 (2007): 25-48.

Sadeharju, K., et al. "Maternal antibodies in breast milk protect the child from enterovirus infections." Pediatrics 119.5 (2007): 941-46.

Salazar-Lindo, E., et al. "Effectiveness and safety of Lactobacillus LB in the treatment of mild acute diarrhea in children." J.Pediatr.Gastroenterol. Nutr. 44.5 (2007): 571-76.

SanGiovanni, J. P., et al. "The relationship of dietary lipid intake and age-related macular degeneration in a case-control study: AREDS Report No. 20." Arch.Ophthalmol. 125.5 (2007): 671-79.

Satter, E. M. "The feeding relationship." J.Am.Diet.Assoc. 86.3 (1986): 352-56.

Scarmeas, N., et al. "Mediterranean diet, Alzheimer disease, and vascular mediation." Arch.Neurol. 63.12 (2006): 1709-17.

Schweizer, H. P. "Triclosan: a widely used biocide and its link to antibiotics." FEMS Microbiol.Lett. 202.1 (2001): 1-7.

Shaw, D. "Risks or remedies? Safety aspects of herbal remedies in the UK." J.R.Soc.Med. 91.6 (1998): 294-96.

Shekelle, P., et al. "Effect of the supplemental use of antioxidants vitamin C, vitamin E, and coenzyme Q10 for the prevention and treatment of cancer." Evid.Rep.Technol.Assess.(Summ.).75 (2003): 1-3.

Shekelle, P., S. Morton, and M. L. Hardy. "Effect of supplemental antioxidants vitamin C, vitamin E, and coenzyme Q10 for the prevention and treatment of cardiovascular disease." Evid.Rep.Technol.Assess. (Summ.).83 (2003): 1-3.

Staruchova, M., et al. "Importance of diet in protection against oxidative damage." Neuro.Endocrinol.Lett. 27 Suppl 2 (2006): 112-15.

---. "Importance of diet in protection against oxidative damage." Neuro. Endocrinol.Lett. 27 Suppl 2 (2006): 112-15.

Toden, S., et al. "Differential effects of dietary whey, casein and soya on colonic DNA damage and large bowel SCFA in rats fed diets low and high in resistant starch." Br.J.Nutr. 97.3 (2007): 535-43.

Trojian, T. H., K. Mody, and P. Chain. "Exercise and colon cancer: primary and secondary prevention." Curr.Sports Med.Rep. 6.2 (2007): 120-24.

Varraso, R., et al. "Prospective study of dietary patterns and chronic obstructive pulmonary disease among US men." Thorax (2007).

Wang, H., et al. "The identification of antioxidants in dark soy sauce." Free Radic. Res. 41.4 (2007): 479-88.

Waser, M., et al. "Inverse association of farm milk consumption with asthma and allergy in rural and suburban populations across Europe." Clin. Exp.Allergy 37.5 (2007): 661-70.

Yaffe, K., et al. "Glycosylated hemoglobin level and development of mild cognitive impairment or dementia in older women." J.Nutr.Health Aging 10.4 (2006): 293-95.

Yazdankhah, S. P., et al. "Triclosan and antimicrobial resistance in bacteria: an overview." Microb.Drug Resist. 12.2 (2006): 83-90.

Yokoyama, M., et al. "Effects of eicosapentaenoic acid on major coronary events in hypercholesterolaemic patients (JELIS): a randomised open-label, blinded endpoint analysis." Lancet 369.9567 (2007): 1090-98.

Websites

www.stress.org/problem.htm

Snapshots

I hope you enjoyed and found some humor in the SNAPSHOTS cartoons found throughout this book.   For more laughs, SNAPSHOTS: The Big Picture, by Jason Love, is available at www.Amazon.com and/or check out www.jasonlove.com.

Notes